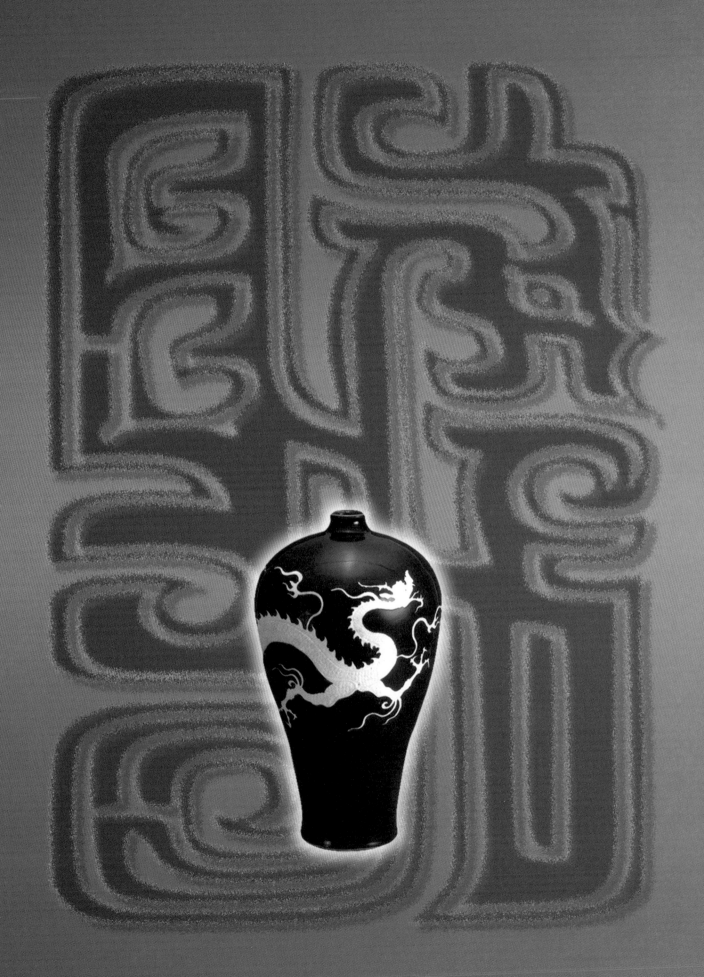

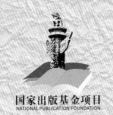

国家出版基金项目

NATIONAL PUBLICATION FOUNDATION

中华医药卫生

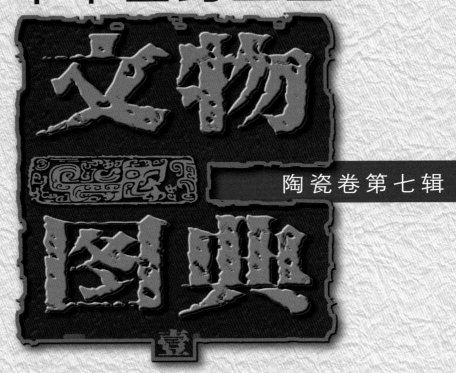

陶瓷卷第七辑

主　编　李经纬　梁　峻　刘学春

总主译　白永权

主　译　范晓晖　温　睿

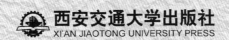

西安交通大学出版社

XI'AN JIAOTONG UNIVERSITY PRESS

图书在版编目（CIP）数据

中华医药卫生文物图典 . 1. 陶瓷卷 . 第 7 辑 . / 李经纬、

梁峻，刘学春主编 . — 西安：西安交通大学出版社，2016.12

ISBN 978-7-5605-7034-1

Ⅰ . ①中… Ⅱ . ①李… ②梁… ③刘… Ⅲ . ①中国医药学—

古代陶瓷—中国—图录 Ⅳ . ① R-092 ② K870.2

中国版本图书馆 CIP 数据核字（2015）第 013562 号

书　　名　中华医药卫生文物图典（一）陶瓷卷第七辑

主　　编　李经纬　梁　峻　刘学春

责任编辑　郭泉泉

出版发行　西安交通大学出版社

　　　　　（西安市兴庆南路 10 号　邮政编码 710049）

网　　址　http://www.xjtupress.com

电　　话　（029）82668805 82668502（医学分社）

　　　　　（029）82668315（总编办）

传　　真　（029）82668280

印　　刷　中煤地西安地图制印有限公司

开　　本　889mm×1194mm　1/16　印张　28.75　字数　470 千字

版次印次　2017 年 12 月第 1 版　2017 年 12 月第 1 次印刷

书　　号　ISBN 978-7-5605-7034-1

定　　价　980.00 元

读者购书、书店添货、如发现印装质量问题，请通过以下方式联系、调换。

订购热线：（029）82665248　（029）82665249

投稿热线：（029）82668805　（029）82668502

读者信箱：medpress@126.com

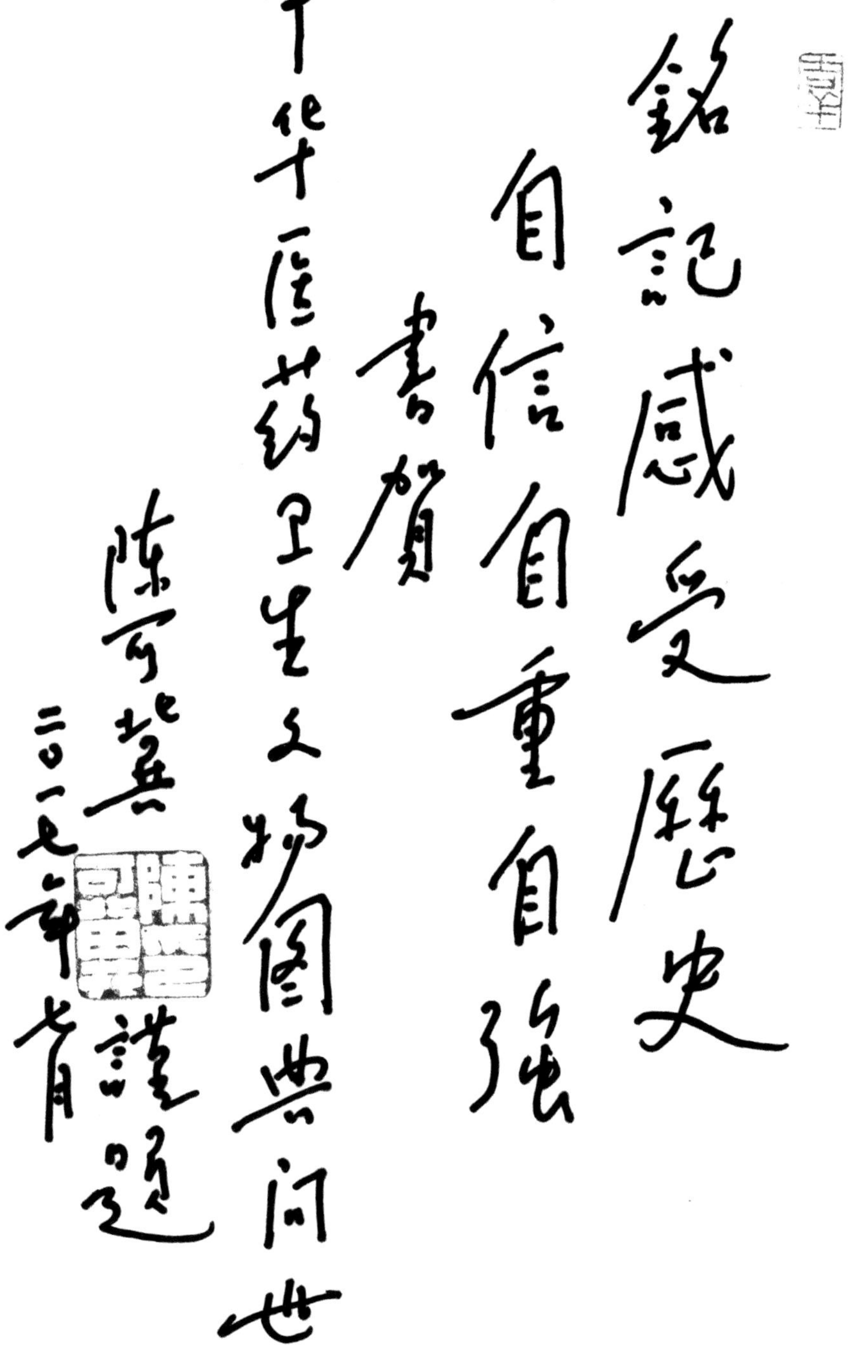

銘記感受歷史

自信自重自強自強

書賀

中華醫藥衛生文物圖典問世

陳可冀 謹題

二〇二〇年春

陈可冀　中国科学院院士、国医大师

精修醫藥衛生文物

圖典功著當代

深究岐黃學術思想

淵源惠澤千秋

中華醫藥衛生文物圖典出版誌慶

丁酉孟秋　孫光榮　敬題於北京

孙光荣　国医大师

中華醫藥衛生文物圖典出版

彰顯中醫藥文化精神

體現中醫藥歷史價值

歲次丁酉夏　王琦

王琦　国医大师

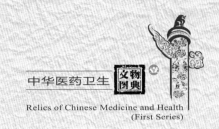

中华医药卫生

Relies of Chinese Medicine and Health
(First Series)

中华医药卫生文物图典（一）
丛书编撰委员会

主　编　李经纬　梁　峻　刘学春

副主编　廖　果　吴鸿洲　康兴军　和中浚　刘小斌　杨金生

　　　　　郑怀林　徐江雁　白建疆　黄　煌

编　委　李洪晓　梁永宣　王强虎　董树平　马　健　王　霞

　　　　　张雅宗　朱德明　包哈申　张建青　郑　蓉　庄乾竹

　　　　　李宏红　刘哲峰　王宏才　陈润东

总主译　白永权

主　译　陈向京　聂文信　范晓晖　温　睿　赵永生　杜彦龙

　　　　　吉　乐　李小棉　郭　梦　陈　曦

副主译（按姓氏音序排列）

　　　　　董艳云　姜雨孜　李建西　刘　慧　马　健　任宝磊

　　　　　任　萌　任　莹　王　颇　习通源　谢皖吉　徐素云

　　　　　许崇钰　许　梅　詹菊红　赵　菲　邹郝晶

译　者（按姓氏音序排列）

迟征宇　邓　甜　付一豪　高　琛　高　媛　郭　宁

韩　蕾　何宗昌　胡勇强　黄　鋆　蒋新蕾　康晓薇

李静波　刘雅恬　刘妍萌　鲁显生　马　月　牛笑语

唐云鹏　唐臻娜　田　多　铁红玲　佟健一　王　晨

王　丹　王　栋　王　丽　王　媛　王慧敏　王梦杰

王仙先　吴耀均　席　慧　肖国强　许子洋　闫红贤

杨姣姣　姚　晔　张　阳　张　鋆　张继飞　张梦原

张晓谦　赵　欣　赵亚力　郑　青　郑艳华　朱江嵩

朱瑛培

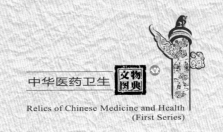

本册编撰委员会

主　编　李经纬　梁　峻　刘学春

副主编　廖　果　吴鸿洲　康兴军　和中浚　刘小斌　杨金生
　　　　郑怀林　徐江雁　白建疆　黄　煌

编　委　李洪晓　梁永宣　王强虎　董树平　马　健　王　霞
　　　　张雅宗　朱德明　包哈申　张建青　郑　蓉　庄乾竹
　　　　李宏红　刘哲峰　王宏才　陈润东

总主译　白永权

主　译　范晓晖　温　睿

副主译　任　萌　佟建一

译　者　朱瑛培　王　栋　唐云鹏　赵　菲　马　月

丛书策划委员会

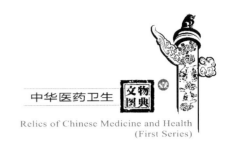

中华医药卫生 文物图典

Relics of Chinese Medicine and Health
(First Series)

序 言

　　探索天、地、人运动变化规律以及"气化物生"过程的相互关系，是人类永恒的课题。宇宙不可逆，地球不可逆，人生不可逆业已成为共识。天地造化形成自然，人类活动构成文化。文物既是文化的载体，又是物化的历史，还是文明的见证。

　　追求健康长寿是人类共同的夙愿。中华民族之所以繁衍昌盛，健康文化起了巨大的推动作用。由于古人谋求生存发展、应对环境变化产生的智慧，大多反映在以医药卫生为核心的健康文化之中，所以，习总书记说："中医药学是中国古代科学的瑰宝，也是打开中华文明宝库的钥匙"。

　　秉持文化大发展、大繁荣理念，中国中医科学院李经纬、梁峻等为负责人的科研团队在完成科技部"国家重点医药卫生文物收集调研和保护"课题获 2005 年度中华中医药学会科技二等奖基础上，又资鉴"夏商周断代工程""中华文明探源工程"等相关考古成果，用有重要价值的新出土文物置换原拍摄质量较差的文物，适当补充民族医药文物，共精选收载 5000 余件。经西安交通大学出版社申报，《中华医药卫生文物图典（一）》（以下简称《图典》）于 2013 年获得了国家出版基金的资助，并经专业翻译团队翻译，使《图典》得以面世。

　　文物承载的信息多元丰富，发掘解读其中蕴藏的智慧并非易事。 医药卫生文物更具有特殊性，除文物的一般属性外，还承载着传统医学发展史迹与促进健康的信息。运用历史唯物主义观察发掘文物信息，善于从生活文物中领悟卫生信息，才能准确解读其功能，也才能诠释其在民生健康中的历史作用，收到以古鉴今之效果。"历史是现实的根源"，任何一个民族都不能割断历史，史料都包含在文化中。"文化是民族的血脉，是人民的精神家园"，文化繁荣才能实现中华民族的伟大复兴。值本《图典》付梓之际，用"梳理文化之脉，必获健康之果"作为序言并和作者、读者共勉！

中央文史研究馆馆员
中国工程院院士　　王永炎

丁酉年仲夏

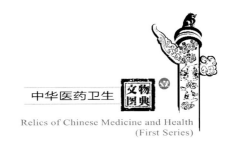

前 言

　　文化是相对自然的概念，是考古界常用词汇。文物是文化的重要组成部分，既是文明的物证，又是物化的历史。狭义医药卫生文物是疾病防治模式语境下的解读，而广义医药卫生文物则是躯体、心态、环境适应三维健康模式下的诠释。中华民族是56个民族组成的多元一体大家庭，中华医药卫生文物当然包括各民族的健康文化遗存。

　　天地造化如造山、板块漂移、气候变迁、生物起源进化等形成自然。气化物生莫贵于人，即整个生物进化的最高成果是人类自身。广义而言，人类生存思维留下的痕迹即物质财富和精神财富总和构成文化，其一般的物化形式是视觉感知的文物、文献、胜迹等。其中质变标志明晰的文化如文字、文物、城市、礼仪等可称作文明。从唯物史观视角观察，狭义文化即精神财富，尤其体现人类精、气、神状态的事项，其本质也具有特殊物质属性，如量子也具有波粒二相性，这种粒子也是物质，无非运动方式特殊而已。现代所谓可重复验证的"科学"，事实上也是从文化中分离出来的事项，因此也是一种特殊文化形式。追求健康长寿是人类共同的夙愿。中华民族之所以繁衍昌盛，是因为健康文化异彩纷呈。中华优秀传统医药文化之所以博大精深，是因为其原创思维博大、格物致知精深，所以，习总书记说："中医药学是中国古代科学的瑰宝，也是打开中华文明宝库的钥匙"。

文化既反映时代、地域、民族分布、生产资料来源、技术水平等信息，又反映人类认知水平和生存智慧。发掘解读文物、文献中蕴藏的健康知识和灵动智慧，首先是从事健康工作者的责任和义务。《易经》设有"观"卦，人类作为观察者，不仅要积极收藏展陈文物，而且要善于捕捉文物倾诉的信息，汲取养分，启迪思维，收到古为今用之效果。墨子三表法，首先一表即"本之于古者圣王之事"，也是强调古代史实的重要性。"历史是现实的根源"，现实是未来的基础。任何一个国家、地区、民族都不能割断历史、忽略基础，这个基础就是文化。"文化是民族的血脉，是人民的精神家园"。文化繁荣才能驱动各项事业发展，才能实现中华民族的伟大复兴。

人类从类人猿分化出来。"禄丰古猿禄丰种"是云南禄丰发现的类人猿化石，距今七八百万年。距今 200 万年前人类进入旧石器时代，直立行走，打制石器产生工具意识，管理火种，是所谓"燧人氏"时代。中国留存有更新世早、中期的元谋、蓝田、北京人等遗址。距今 10 万—5 万年前，人类进入旧石器时代中期，即早期智人阶段，脑容量增加，和欧洲、非洲人种相比，原始蒙古人种颧骨前突等，是所谓"伏羲氏"时代。中国发现的马坝、长阳、丁村人等较典型。距今 5 万—1 万年前，人类进入旧石器时代晚期，即晚期智人阶段，细石器、骨角器等遍布全国，山顶洞、柳江、资阳人等较典型。

中石器时代距今约 1 万年，是旧石器时代向新石器时代的短暂过渡期，弓箭发明，狗被驯化。河南灵井、陕西沙苑遗址等作为代表。距今 1 万—公元前 2600 年前后，人类进入新石器时代，磨光石器、烧制陶器，出现农业村落并饲养家畜，是所谓"神农氏"时代。公元前 7000 年以来，在甲、骨、陶、石等载体上出现契刻符号、七音阶骨笛乐器等，反映出人文气息趋浓。公元前 6000—公元前 3500 年的老官台、裴李岗、河姆渡、马家浜、仰韶等文化遗址，彰显出先民围绕生存健康问题所做的各种努力。

公元前 4800 年以来，以关中、晋南、豫西为中心形成的仰韶文化，是中原史前文化的重要标志。以半坡、庙底沟类型为典型，自公元前 3500 年走向繁荣，属于锄耕粟黍稻兼营渔猎饲养猪鸡经济方式，彩陶尤其发达。公元前 4400—公元前 3300 年，长江中游的大溪文化，薄胎彩陶和白陶发达。公元前 4300—公元前 2500 年山东丰岛的大汶口文化，红陶为主。公元前 3500 年前后，辽东的红山文化原始宗教发展。公元前 3300 年以来，长江下游由河姆渡、马家浜文化衍续的良渚文化和陇西的马家窑文化、江淮间的薛家岗文化时趋发达。

公元前 2600—公元前 2000 年，黄河中下游龙山文化群形成，冶铸铜器，制作玉器，土坯、石灰、夯筑技术开始应用。公元前 2697 年，轩辕战败炎帝（有说其后裔）、蚩尤而为黄帝纪元元年。黄帝西巡访贤，"至岐见岐伯，引载而归，访于治道"。其引归地"溱洧襟带于前，梅泰环拱于后"，即今河南新密市古城寨。岐黄答问，构建《黄帝内经》健康知识体系，中华文明从关注民生健康起步。颛顼改革宗教，神职人员出现；帝喾修身节用，帝尧和合百国，舜同律度量衡，大禹疏导治水，中华民族不断繁衍昌盛。

公元前 2070 年，禹之子启以豫西晋南为中心建立夏王朝，二里头青铜文化为其特征，半地穴、窑洞、地面建筑并存。饮食卫生器具、酒器增多。朱砂安神作用在宫殿应用。公元前 1600 年，商灭夏。偃师商城设有铸铜作坊。公元前 1300 年，盘庚迁殷，使用甲骨文。武丁时期青铜浑铸、分铸并存。公元前 1056 年，相传周"文王被殷纣拘于羑里，演《周易》，成六十四卦"。公元前 1046 年，武王克商建周，定都镐京。青铜器始铸长篇铭文，周原发掘出微型甲骨文字。公元前 770 年，平王东迁。虢国铸铜柄铁剑。公元前 753 年，秦国设置史官。公元前 707 年出现蝗灾、公元前 613 年出现"哈雷彗星"，均被孔子载入《春秋》。公元前 221 年，秦始皇统一中国，多元一体民族大家庭形成，中华医药卫生文物异彩纷呈。

中国是治史大国，历来重视发展文化博物事业，1955 年成立卫生部中医研究院时就设置医史研究室，1982 年中国医史文献研究所成立时复建中国医史博物馆研究收藏展陈文物。2000—2003 年，经王永炎院士、姚乃礼院长等呼吁，科技部批准立项，由李经纬、梁峻为负责人的团队完成"国家重点医药卫生文物收集调研和保护"项目任务，受到科技部项目验收组专家的高度评价，获中华中医药学会科技进步二等奖。2013 年，在国家出版基金资助下，课题组对部分文物重新拍摄或必要置换、充实民族医药文物后，由西安交通大学出版社编辑、组聘国内一流翻译团队英译说明文字付梓，受到国家中医药博物馆筹备工作领导小组和办公室的高度重视。

"物以类聚"，《图典》主要依据文物质地、种类分为 9 卷，计有陶瓷，金属，纸质，竹木，玉石、织品及标本，壁画石刻及遗址，少数民族文物，其他，备考等卷。同卷下主要根据历史年代或小类分册设章。每卷下的历史时段不求统一。遵循上述规则将《图典》划分为21册，总计收载文物5000余件。对每件文物的描述，除质地、规格、馆藏等基本要素外，重点描述其在民生健康中的作用。对少数暂不明确的事项在括号中注明待考。对引自各博物馆的材料除在文物后列出馆藏外，还在书后再次统一列出馆名或参考书目，以充分尊重其馆藏权，也同时维护本典作者的引用权。

21世纪，围绕人类健康的生命科学将飞速发展，但科学离不开文化，文化离不开文物。发掘文物承载的信息为现实服务，谨引用横渠先生四言之两语："为天地立心，为生民立命"，既作为编撰本《图典》之宗旨，也是我们践行国家"一带一路"倡议的具体努力。希冀通过本《图典》的出版发行，教育国人，提振中华民族精神；走向世界，为人类健康事业贡献力量。

李经纬　梁峻　刘学春

2017年6月于北京

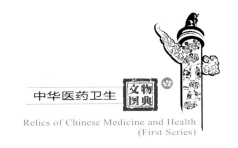

中华医药卫生 文物图典

Relics of Chinese Medicine and Health
(First Series)

目 录

3

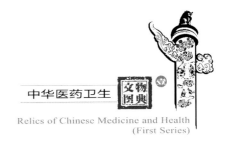

中华医药卫生　文物图典

Relics of Chinese Medicine and Health
(First Series)

Contents

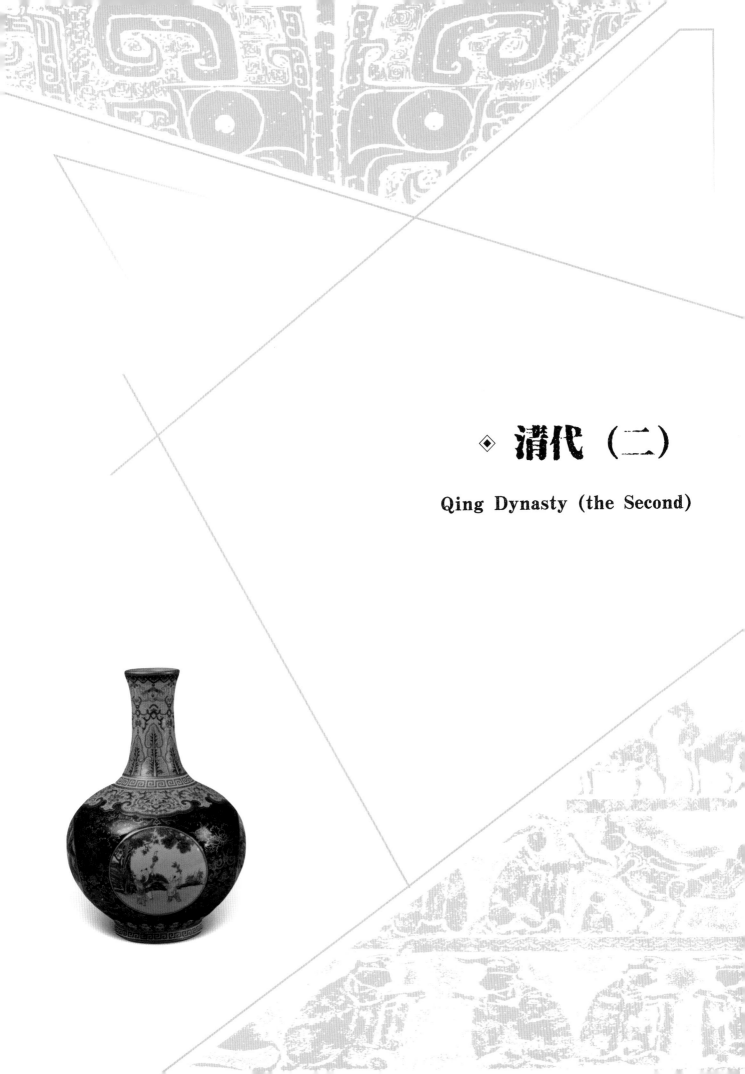

◇ **清代（二）**

Qing Dynasty (the Second)

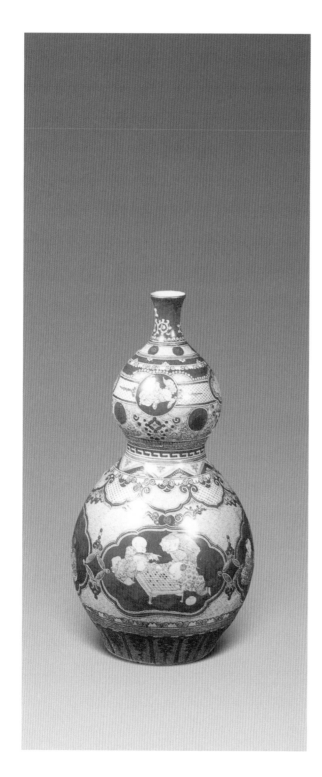

五彩弈棋纹葫芦瓷瓶

清

瓷质

通高 36 厘米

Gourd-shaped Porcelain Vase with Chess Playing Scene in Famille Verte Glaze

Qing Dynasty

Porcelain

Height 36 cm

瓶呈葫芦状，通体白釉红绿彩装饰。弈棋纹绘于
下腹部，图中有两小童围在棋盘旁对弈，另一位
在一边指指点点，出谋划策，旁有一老者，在弓
腰观看。

日本石川县立美术馆藏

The gourd-shaped vase glazed white has red and
green decorations. In the lower part there are two
children playing Chinese chess, and beside them
there are another child gesticulating to give advice
and an old man bending down and watching.
Preserved in Ishikawa Prefectural Museum of Art

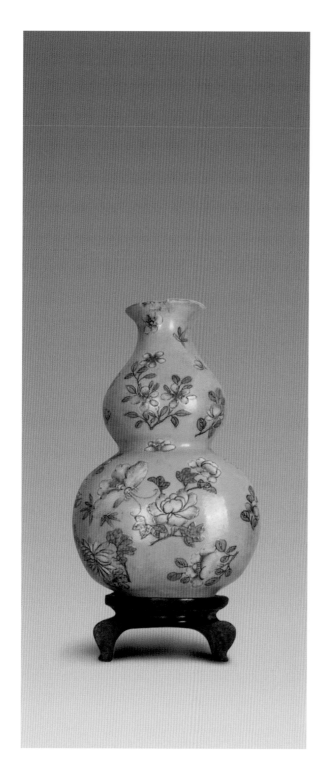

绿彩半葫芦挂瓶

清

瓷质

上腹径 6.5 厘米，下腹径 9.8 厘米，通高 16 厘米

Half-gourd-shaped Wall Bottle Glazed Green

Qing Dynasty

Porcelain

Upper Belly Diameter 6.5 cm/ Lower Belly Diameter 9.8 cm/ Height 16 cm

半葫芦形。该瓶为绿釉，瓶面工笔粉蝶桃
花图案，画工精细。为盛药器具。1957 年
入藏。保存基本完好。

中华医学会 / 上海中医药大学医史博物馆

The half-gourd-shaped bottle glazed green
is exquisitely painted with a pink butterfly
and peach blossoms in fine brushwork. It
was used to store medicines. The bottle was
collected by the museum in 1957 and is still
in good condition.

Preserved in Chinese Medical Association/
Museum of Chinese Medicine, Shanghai
University of Traditional Chinese Medicine

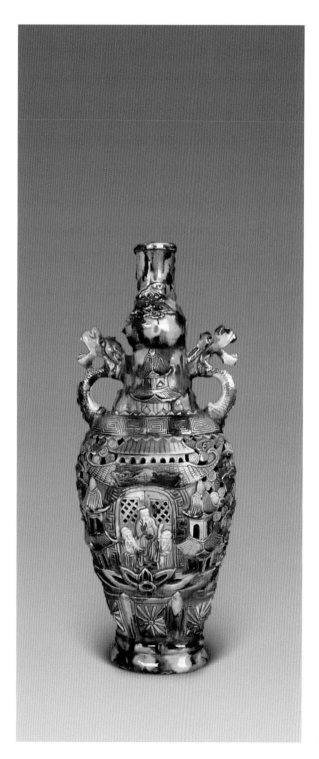

五彩瓷瓶

清

瓷质

口外径 3.6 厘米，口内径 2.9 厘米，宽 14.5 厘米，
厚 9.5 厘米，高 35 厘米

Famille Verte Porcelain Vase

Qing Dynasty

Porcelain

Mouth Outer Diameter 3.6 cm/ Mouth Inner
Diameter 2.9 cm/ Width 14.5 cm/ Thickness 9.5 cm/
Height 35 cm

葫芦形。该藏直口圈足双龙耳，通身镂雕有卷云、亭台楼阁和福禄寿图案。底有"大清康熙年制"款识。为工艺品。工艺较好。1956 年入藏，保存基本完好。

中华医学会 / 上海中医药大学医史博物馆

The gourd-shaped handicraft has a verical mouth, two dragon-shaped handles on both sides, and a ring foot. The whole body is decorated with pierced curved clouds, pavilions and patterns representing good fortune, prosperity and longevity. The base is inscribed with six Chinese words "Da Qing Kang Xi Nian Zhi" (made during Kangxi Reign of the Qing Dynasty). The bottle is fine in workmanship. It was collected by the museum in 1956 and is basically in good condition. Preserved in Chinese Medical Association/ Museum of Chinese Medicine, Shanghai University of Traditional Chinese Medicine

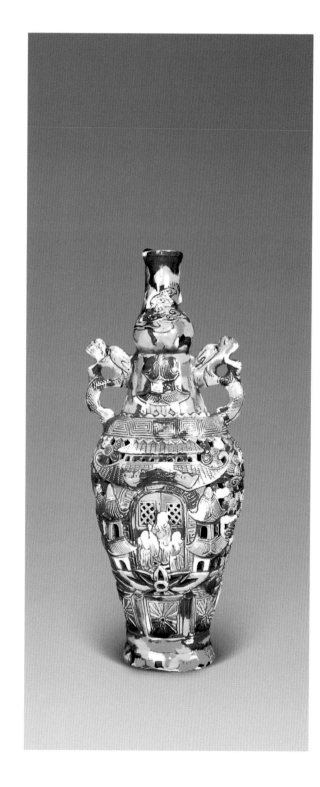

五彩瓷瓶

清

瓷质

口外径3.6厘米，口内径2.9厘米，宽14.5厘米，
厚9.5厘米，高36厘米

Famille Verte Porcelain Vase

Qing Dynasty

Porcelain

Mouth Outer Diameter 3.6 cm/ Mouth Inner
Diameter 2.9 cm/ Width 14.5 cm/ Thickness 9.5
cm/ Height 36 cm

葫芦形。该藏直口圈足双龙耳，通身镂雕有卷云、亭台楼阁和福禄寿图案。底有"大清康熙年制"款识。为工艺品。工艺较好。1956 年入藏，保存基本完好。

中华医学会 / 上海中医药大学医史博物馆

The gourd-shaped handicraft has a vertical mouth, two dragon-shaped handles on both sides, and a ring foot. The whole body is decorated with pierced curved clouds, pavilions and patterns of good fortune, prosperity and longevity. The base is inscribed with six Chinese words "Da Qing Kang Xi Nian Zhi" (made during Kangxi Reign of the Qing Dynasty). The bottle is fine in workmanship. It was collected by the museum in 1956 and is basically in good condition.

Preserved in Chinese Medical Association/ Museum of Chinese Medicine, Shanghai University of Traditional Chinese Medicine

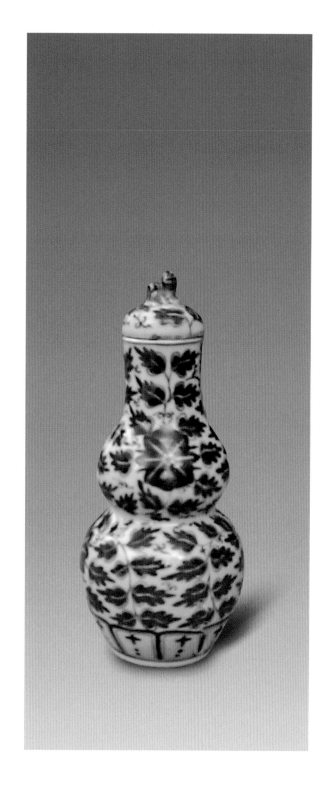

葫芦瓶

清

瓷质

口径 4.4 厘米，上腹径 7.7 厘米，下腹径 10.1 厘米，

底径 5.8 厘米，通高 22.4 厘米

Gourd-shaped Bottle

Qing Dynasty

Porcelain

Mouth Diameter 4.4 cm/ Upper Belly Diameter

7.7 cm/ Lower Belly Diameter 10.1 cm/ Bottom

Diameter 5.8 cm/ Height 22.4 cm

葫芦形。该藏青花釉，平底，敞口，带盖，
工艺精细，造型美观。为盛药器具。1959 年
入藏，保存基本完好。

中华医学会 / 上海中医药大学医史博物馆

The gourd-shaped bottle has a flared mouth,
a flat bottom, and a lid. The blue-and-white
bottle was once used for keeping medicines.
It is exquisite and beautifully shaped. The
bottle was collected by the museum in 1959
and is basically in good condition.

Preserved in Chinese Medical Association/
Museum of Chinese Medicine, Shanghai
University of Traditional Chinese Medicine

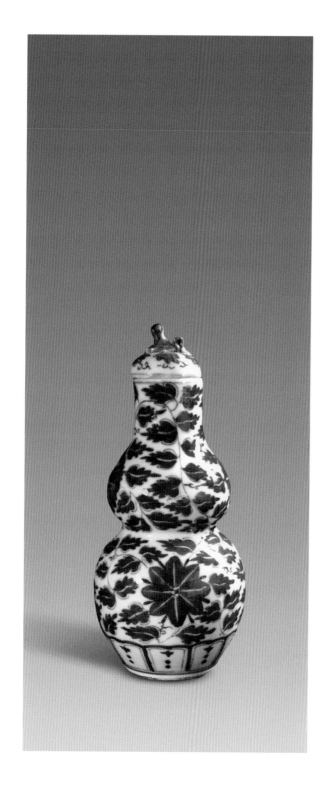

青花缠枝花纹葫芦药瓶

清

瓷质

底径 20 厘米，通高 34 厘米

Gourd-shaped Medicine Bottle Patterned with Intertwining Branches

Qing Dynasty

Porcelain

Bottom Diameter 20 cm/ Height 34 cm

直口，平沿，平底，有盖，盖上塑一虎钮。
青花缠枝花纹繁而不乱。

上海中医药博物馆藏

The medicine bottle has a cvertical mouth, a flat rim, a flat bottom, and a lid with a tiger-shaped knob. It is decorated with blue-and-white intertwining flower branches which are numerous and neatly arranged.

Preserved in Shanghai Museum of Traditional Chinese Medicine

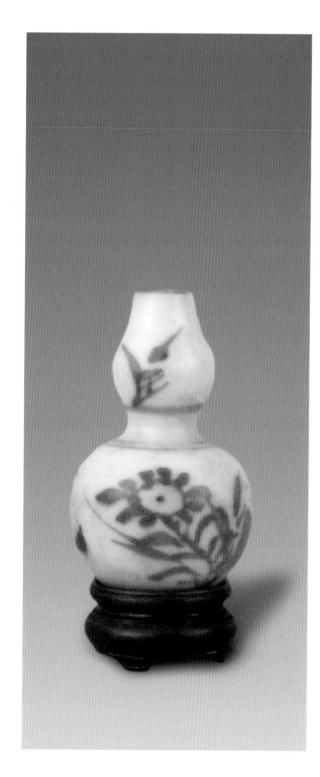

葫芦瓶

清

瓷质

口径 1.1 厘米，上腹径 1.8 厘米，下腹径 3.2 厘米，
通高 5.1 厘米

Gourd-shaped Bottle

Qing Dynasty

Porcelain

Mouth Diameter 1.1 cm/ Upper Belly Diameter
1.8 cm/ Lower Belly diameter 3.2 cm/ Height 5.1 cm

葫芦形。该藏青花釉，绘花草 图案，平底，直口，小巧玲珑，造型美观。为盛药器具。1955 年入藏，保存基本完好。

中华医学会 / 上海中医药大学医史博物馆

The gourd-shaped bottle has a vertical mouth and a flat bottom. It is painted with blue-and-white flower and grass motifs. The bijou bottle has beautiful modelling. It was used for keeping medicines. The bottle was collected in 1955 and is basically in good condition.

Preserved in Chinese Medical Association/ Museum of Chinese Medicine, Shanghai University of Traditional Chinese Medicine

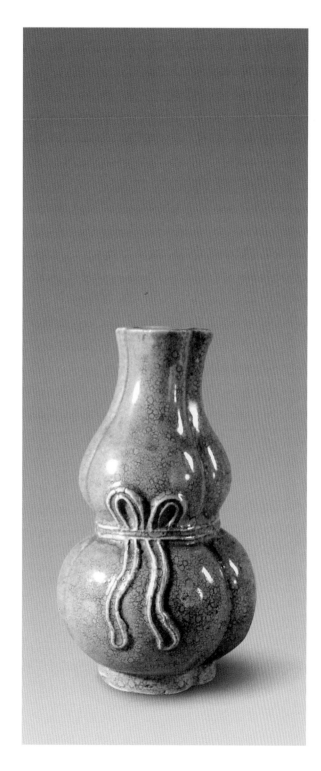

三口葫芦瓷瓶

清

瓷质

底径最宽 6 厘米，通高 14 厘米

Triple-mouthed Porcelain Medicine Bottle

Qing Dynasty

Porcelain

Maximum Bottom Diameter 6 cm/ Height 14 cm

侈口，长颈，平底，下顶有半圆形三口相连，
内分三腔。葫芦腰部有带系纹。

上海中医药博物馆藏

The gourd-shaped bottle has a flared mouth, a
long neck, and a flat bottom. Its three semicircular
mouths are open into separate cavities. There is a
bowknot motif on the belly.

Preserved in Shanghai Museum of Traditional
Chinese Medicine

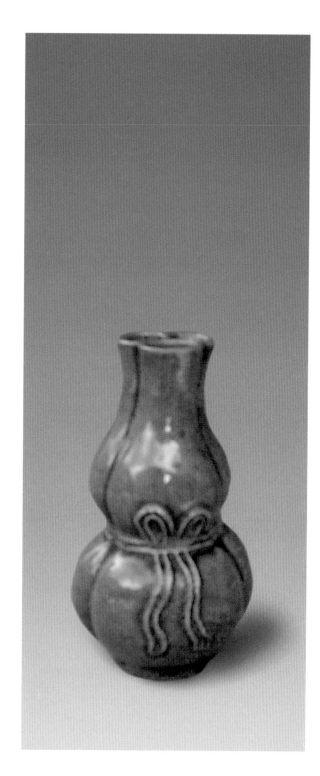

三口葫芦瓶

清

瓷质

口径 3.3 厘米，上腹径 5.3 厘米，下腹径 6.7 厘米，
底径 4.1 厘米，通高 11.3 厘米

Triple-mouthed Gourd-shaped Bottle

Qing Dynasty

Porcelain

Mouth Diameter 3.3 cm/ Upper Belly Diameter 5.3 cm/

Lower Belly Diameter 6.7 cm/ Bottom Diameter 4.1 cm/

Height 11.3 cm

葫芦形。该藏蓝绿釉，平底，口分三腔，腰部浮雕系绳蝴蝶节状，工艺精细，造型别致。为盛药器具。1955 年入藏，保存基本完好。

中华医学会 / 上海中医药大学医史博物馆

The gourd-shaped bottle, which is coated with bluish green glaze, has three separate mouths, a flat bottom, and a relief design of bowknot on the belly. The exquisite bottle with special modelling was used for keeping medicines. It was collected by the museum in 1955 and is basically in good condition.
Preserved in Chinese Medical Association/ Museum of Chinese Medicine, Shanghai University of Traditional Chinese Medicine

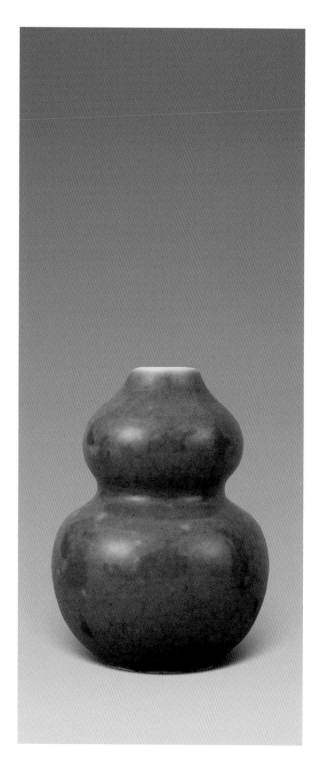

葫芦瓶

清

瓷质

口径1.6厘米，上腹径3.3厘米，下腹径4.4厘米，

通高5.7厘米

Gourd-shaped Bottle

Qing Dynasty

Porcelain

Mouth Diameter 1.6 cm/ Upper Belly Diameter

3.3 cm/ Lower Belly Diameter 4.4 cm/ Height 5.7 cm

葫芦形。该藏通身天蓝釉，平底直口，工艺精巧，造型美观。为盛药器具。1954 年入藏，保存基本完好。

中华医学会 / 上海中医药大学医史博物馆

The gourd-shaped bottle, which was used for keeping medicines, has a straight mouth and a flat base. The exquisite and beautifully shaped bottle is covered with sky blue glaze all over. It was collected by the museum in 1954 and is basically in good condition.

Preserved in Chinese Medical Association/ Museum of Chinese Medicine, Shanghai University of Traditional Chinese Medicine

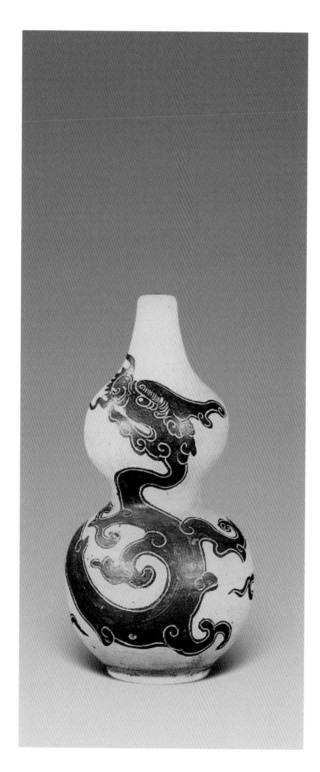

蟠龙葫芦药瓶

清

瓷质

口径 4 厘米，底径 8 厘米，高 18 厘米

Medicine Bottle with Coiled Dragons

Qing Dynasty

Porcelain

Mouth Diameter 4 cm/ Bottom Diameter 8 cm/

Height 18 cm

葫芦形。弇口，平沿，平底。酱黄色釉，饰以蟠龙图案。

上海中医药博物馆藏

The gourd-shaped bottle has a small mouth, a flat rim, and a flat bottom. It is covered with brown glaze and painted with coiled dragon patterns.

Preserved in Shanghai Museum of Traditional Chinese Medicine

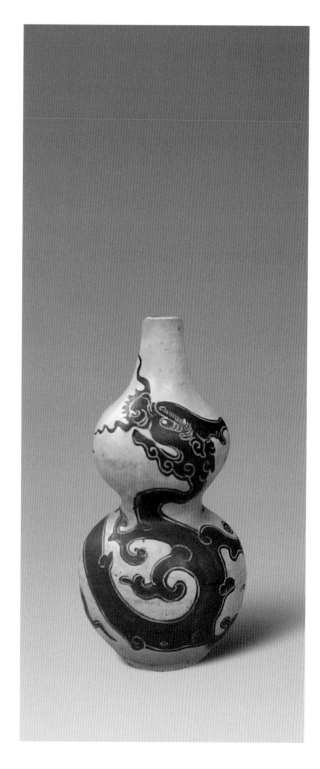

葫芦瓶

清

瓷质

口径 3.1 厘米，上腹径 9.9 厘米，下腹径 1.3 厘米，底径 7.3 厘米，通高 24.4 厘米

Gourd-shaped Bottle

Qing Dynasty

Porcelain

Mouth Diameter 3.1 cm/ Upper Belly Diameter 9.9 cm/ Lower Belly diameter 1.3 cm/ Bottom Diameter 7.3 cm/ Height 24.4 cm

葫芦形。该藏品施白釉底色，上绘黑龙，平底直口，画工精细，造型美观。为盛药器具。1954 年入藏，保存基本完好。

中华医学会 / 上海中医药大学医史博物馆

The gourd-shaped bottle has a vertical mouth and a flat bottom. It is exquisitely painted with a black dragon against the white-glazed background. The bottle, which has exquisite painting work and beautiful modelling. It was used for keeping medicines. It was collected by the museum in 1954 and is basically in good condition.

Preserved in Chinese Medical Association/ Museum of Chinese Medicine, Shanghai University of Traditional Chinese Medicine

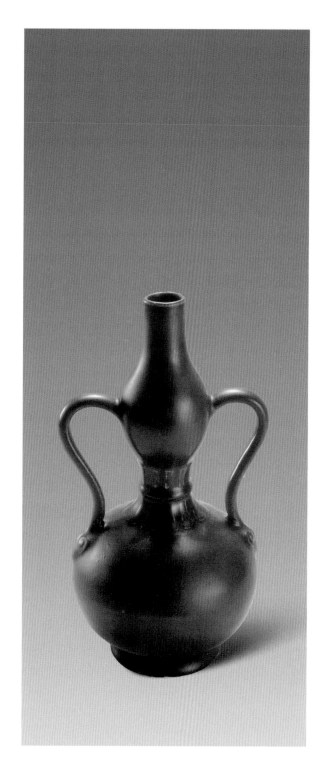

乾隆茶末釉葫芦瓶

清

瓷质

口径 3 厘米，高 26 厘米

Gourd-shaped Vase Glazed Tea-dust Brown, Qianlong Reign

Qing Dynasty

Porcelain

Mouth Diameter 3 cm/ Height 26 cm

瓶为葫芦形，束腰部分有凸起的纹饰带，两
节腹间置细长对称的双曲柄，圈足底，胎灰
黑，满施茶末色釉，釉有细细的流淌痕迹。
底钤三行方形阴文"大清乾隆年制"印，为
景德镇官窑瓷器。瓶为传世品。

扬州博物馆藏

The gourd-shaped vase, which has been handed
down for generations, has relief patterns of
ribbons around the waist; a pair of thin, long
and curved handles on both sides, and a ring
foot. Its cinereous body is covered with tea-dust
brown glaze, which shows small fluid traces.
The bottom of the vase is inscribed with three
lines of Chinese words "Da Qing Qian Long
Nian Zhi" (made during Qianlong Reign of
the Qing Dynasty) in intaglio. The artifact was
made in a governmental kiln in Jingdezhen,
Jiangxi Province.

Preserved in Yangzhou Museum

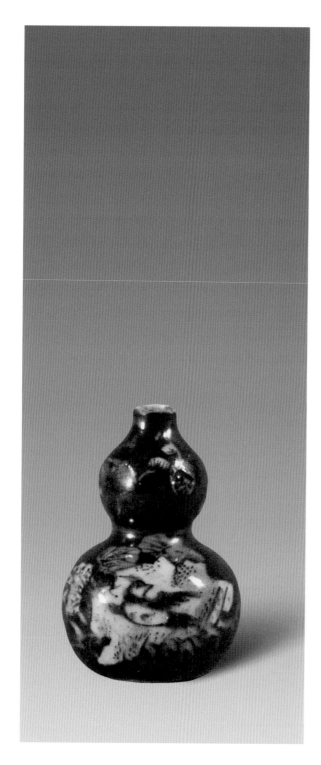

黑釉葫芦小药瓶

清

瓷质

口径 4 厘米，底径 8 厘米，通高 18 厘米

Small Gourd-shaped Medicine Bottle with Black Glaze

Qing Dynasty

Porcelain

Mouth Diameter 4 cm/ Bottom Diameter 8 cm/ Height 18 cm

瓶作葫芦形。口沿有残，平底，酱黑色釉，
饰以飞鸟图案。

上海中医药博物馆藏

The gourd-shaped bottle has a broken mouth
and a flat bottom. It is covered with black glaze
and painted with flying bird patterns.
Preserved in Shanghai Museum of Traditional
Chinese Medicine

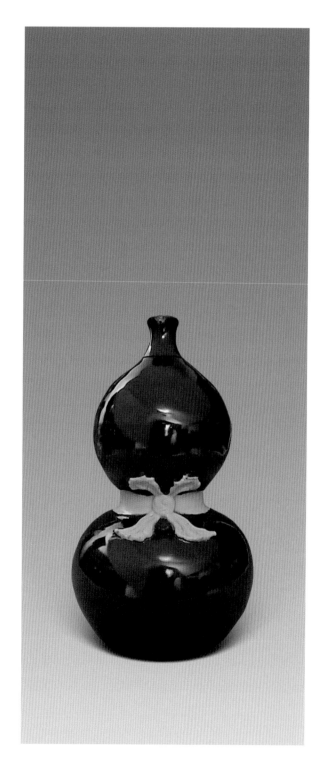

葫芦瓶

清

瓷质

口径 3.1 厘米，上腹径 9.9 厘米，下腹径 13 厘米，底径 7.3 厘米，通高 24.4 厘米

Gourd-shaped Bottle

Qing Dynasty

Porcelain

Mouth Diameter 3.1 cm/ Upper Belly Diameter 9.9 cm/ Lower Belly Diameter 13 cm/ Bottom Diameter 7.3 cm/ Height 24.4 cm

葫芦形。该藏白釉底色，上绘黑龙，平底直口，画工精细，造型美观。为盛药器具。1954 年入藏，保存基本完好。

中华医学会 / 上海中医药大学医史博物馆

The gourd-shaped bottle, which was used for keeping medicines, has a vertical mouth and a flat bottom. It is painted with black dragon patterns against the white-glazed background. There is a relief bowknot motif around its waist. The bottle has exquisite painting work and beautiful modelling. It was collected by the museum in 1954 and is basically in good condition.

Preserved in Chinese Medical Association/ Museum of Chinese Medicine, Shanghai University of Traditional Chinese Medicine

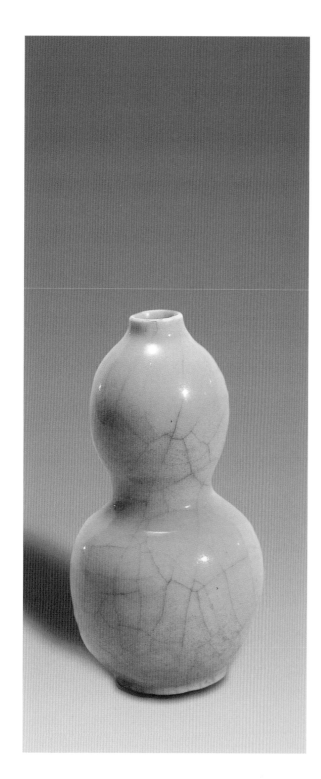

瓷葫芦

清

瓷质

口径 3.2 厘米，腹径 11 厘米，高 21.5 厘米

Gourd-shaped Porcelain Bottle

Qing Dynasty

Porcelain

Mouth Diameter 3.2 cm/ Bottom Diameter 11 cm/

Height 21.5 cm

本品为豆青瓷葫芦，瓷质莹润，釉色淡雅，

大开片。为清乾隆时之佳品。

成都中医药大学中医药传统文化博物馆藏

The bottle is shaped like a gourd. It is
coated with green glaze, with lustrous body
and elegant color, and is heavily crackled.
The bottle was one of the best artworks of
Qianlong Reign of the Qing Dynasty.
Preserved in Museum of Traditional Chinese
Medicine Culture, Chengdu University of
Traditional Chinese Medicine

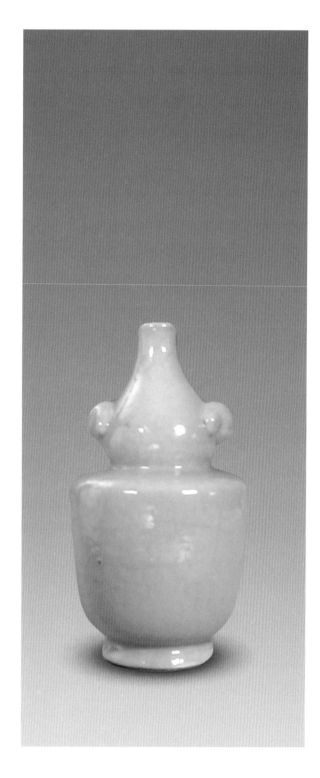

葫芦瓶

清

瓷质

口径 2.4 厘米，上腹径 9 厘米，下腹径 11.1 厘米，

底径 6.5 厘米，通高 19.8 厘米

Gourd-shaped Bottle

Qing Dynasty

Porcelain

Mouth Diameter 2.4 cm/ Upper Belly Diameter

9 cm/ Lower Belly Diameter 11.1 cm/ Bottom

Diameter 6.5 cm/ Height 19.8 cm

葫芦形。该藏品施蓝灰釉，圈足平底直口，肩置双钮，工艺精细，造型美观。为盛药器具。1954 年入藏，保存基本完好。

中华医学会 / 上海中医药大学医史博物馆

The gourd-shaped bottle, which is coated with bluish gray glaze, was used for keeping medicines. It has a vertical mouth, a flat bottom, a ring foot, and two knobs on both sides of the shoulder. The delicate and beautifully modelled bottle was collected by the museum in 1954 and is basically in good condition.

Preserved in Chinese Medical Association/ Museum of Chinese Medicine, Shanghai University of Traditional Chinese Medicine

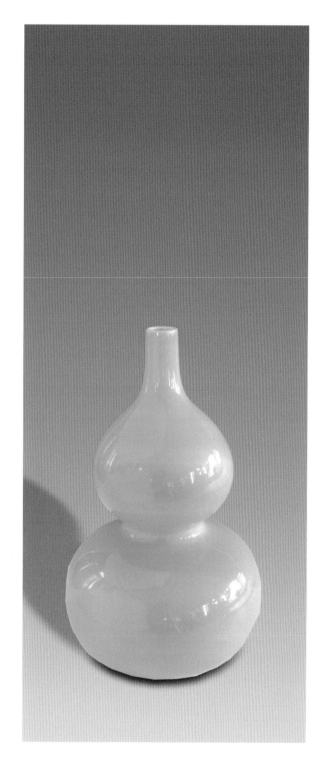

天青釉葫芦瓶

清

瓷质

通高 22 厘米

Gourd-shaped Azure-glazed Vase

Qing Dynasty

Porcelain

Height 22 cm

细口，束腰，上下丰圆腹，卧圈足，全身施天青色釉。底书"大清乾隆年制"六字楷书青花款。该瓶应是产自景德镇乾隆年间的官窑代表作品。

李牧之藏

The vase, which is coated with azure glaze, has a small mouth, a contracted waist, plump upper and lower bellies, and a ring foot. The bottom is inscribed with blue-and-white Chinese words "Da Qing Qian Long Nian Zhi" (made during Qianlong Reign of the Qing Dynasty) in regular script. The vase may be a masterpiece made in a governmental kiln in Jingdezhen during Qianlong Reign.

Collected by Li Muzhi

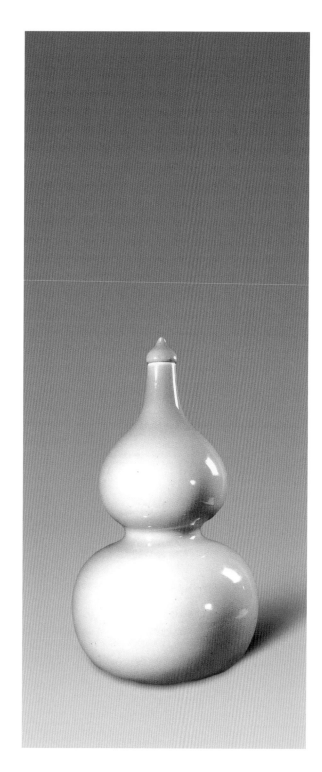

冬青釉葫芦药瓶

清

瓷质

口径 3 厘米，底径 10 厘米，高 35 厘米

Gourd-shaped Holly-glazed Medicine Bottle

Qing Dynasty

Porcelain

Mouth Diameter 3 cm/ Bottom Diameter 10 cm/ Height 35 cm

葫芦形。直口，平沿，圈足，上有盖。底部
中部凹进，敷釉，有 2.5 厘米的款印。

上海中医药博物馆藏

The gourd-shaped medicine bottle has a straight
mouth, a lid, a flat rim, and a ring foot. The
center of the base is concave and glazed, with a
2.5 cm seal.

Preserved in Shanghai Museum of Traditional
Chinese Medicine

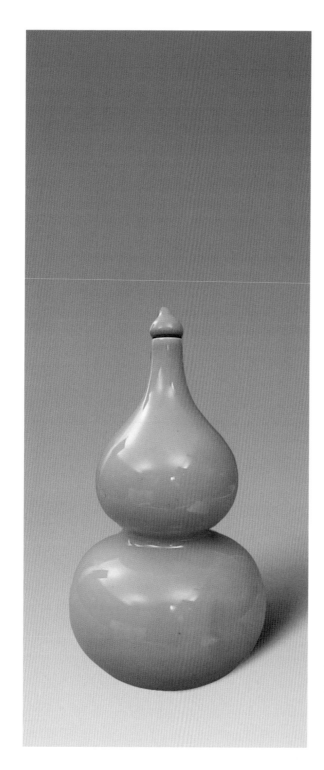

葫芦瓶

清

瓷质

口径 3 厘米，上腹径 14.1 厘米，下腹径 20.6 厘米，底径 11 厘米，通高 35.2 厘米

Gourd-shaped Bottle

Qing Dynasty

Porcelain

Mouth Diameter 3 cm/ Upper Belly Diameter 14.1 cm/ Lower Belly 20.6 cm/ Bottom Diameter 11 cm/ Height 35.2 cm

葫芦形。该藏鹅蛋青釉，釉面光亮无纹饰，平底直口上配盖，盖上有尖钮，制作精细，造型美观。为盛药器具。1952 年入藏，保存基本完好。

中华医学会 / 上海中医药大学医史博物馆

The gourd-shaped bottle, which is coated with glossy goose-egg blue glaze without any pattern, has a vertical mouth, a lid with a pointed knob, and a flat bottom. It was used for keeping medicines. The delicate and beautifully modelled bottle was collected by the museum in 1952 and is basically in good condition.

Preserved in Chinese Medical Association/ Museum of Chinese Medicine, Shanghai University of Traditional Chinese Medicine

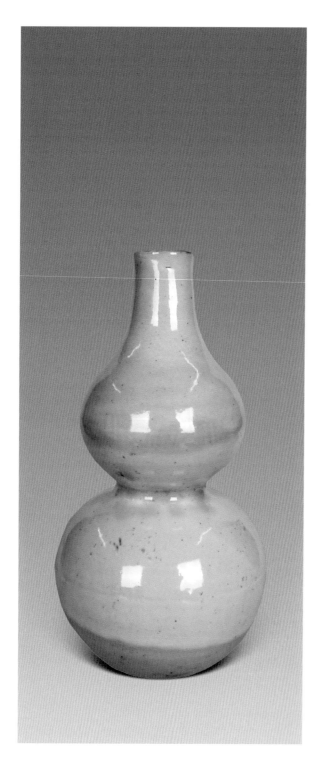

葫芦瓷瓶

清

瓷质

上腹径 10.25 厘米，下腹径 13.6 厘米，通高
25.5 厘米

Gourd-shaped Porcelain Bottle

Qing Dynasty

Porcelain

Upper Belly Diameter 10.25 cm/ Lower Belly
Diameter 13.6 cm/ Height 25.5 cm

葫芦形。该瓶通身施浅灰釉，釉色不匀，表面粗糙，瓷胎有旋纹，瓶底无款识。为盛药器具。1958 年入藏，保存基本完好。

中华医学会 / 上海中医药大学医史博物馆

The gourd-shaped bottle is covered with pale gray glaze, which is uneven and coarse. There are bowstring patterns around the pottery body, but there is no inscription on the bottom. The bottle was used for keeping medicines. It was collected by the museum in 1958 and is basically in good condition.

Preserved in Chinese Medical Association/ Museum of Chinese Medicine, Shanghai University of Traditional Chinese Medicine

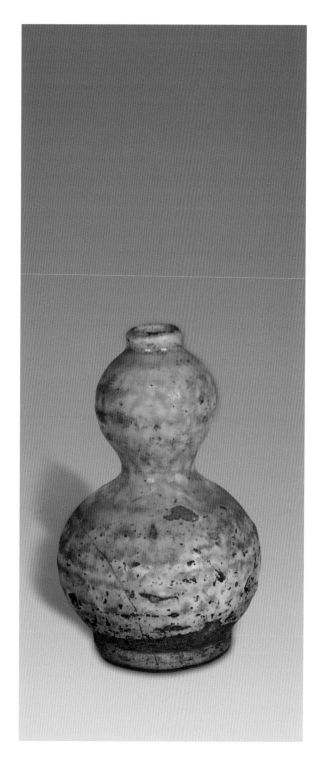

葫芦瓶

清

瓷质

口径 2.65 厘米，上腹径 5.6 厘米，下腹径 9.6 厘米，

通高 14.7 厘米

Gourd-shaped Bottle

Qing Dynasty

Porcelain

Mouth Diameter 2.65 cm/ Upper Belly Diameter

5.6 cm/ Lower Belly Diameter 9.6 cm/ Height

14.7 cm

葫芦形。该藏乳白釉，釉下旋纹明显，底足无釉，圈足平底直口，工艺粗糙，表面凸凹不平。为盛药器具。1956 年入藏，开裂严重，釉面脱落。

中华医学会 / 上海中医药大学医史博物馆

The gourd-shaped bottle has a vertical mouth, a flat bottom, and an unglazed ring foot. The coarse body is covered with milky glaze, under which bowstring patterns can be seen clearly. There is a long crack on the lower part, and parts of the glaze has came off. The bottle, which was used for keeping medicines, was collected by the museum in 1956.

Preserved in Chinese Medical Association/ Museum of Chinese Medicine, Shanghai University of Traditional Chinese Medicine

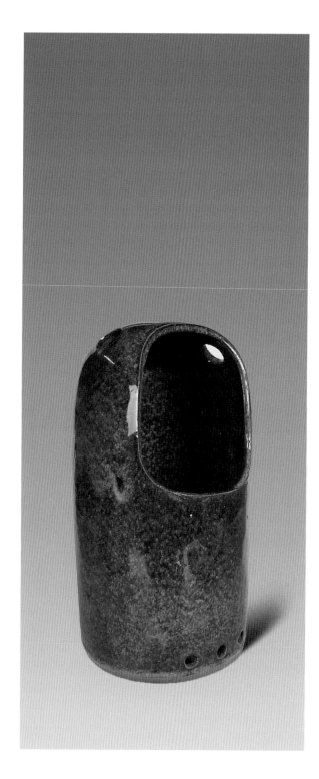

瓷火罐

清

瓷质

直径 16 厘米，通高 29.5 厘米

Porcelain Cupping Jar

Qing Dynasty

Porcelain

Diameter 16 cm/ Height 29.5 cm

圆筒形。该藏外施兰釉，内施酱色釉，上部
开一较大斜口（外径14厘米，内径13厘米），
肩部留有三个气孔（直径2.4厘米），圈足
壁上正面三个孔背面二个孔（孔径1.1厘米），
罐底无釉，有"葛明祥造"款识。为火罐器
具。1957年入藏。

中华医学会 / 上海中医药大学医史博物馆

The cylindrical cupping jar is glazed blue
on the exterior and dark reddish brown on the
interior. On its upper part there is a big sloping
mouth (14 cm in outer diameter and 13 cm in
internal diameter). On its shoulder there are
three holes (2.4 cm in diameter). On the ring
foot wall there are three and two holes (1.1 cm
in diameter for each) on the front side and
the back side, respectively. The unglazed
bottom is inscribed with Chinese words "Ge
Ming Xiang Zao" (made by Ge Mingxiang).
The jar was collected by the museum in
1957.
Preserved in Chinese Medical Association/
Museum of Chinese Medicine, Shanghai
University of Traditional Chinese Medicine

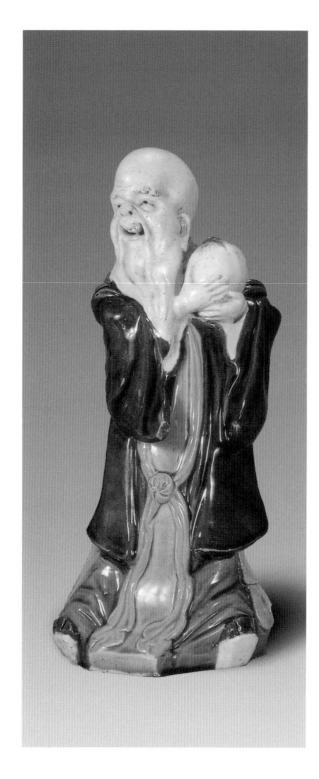

素三彩寿星捧桃像

清

瓷质

通高 28 厘米

Famille Verte Figurine of God of Longevity Holding a Peach

Qing Dynasty

Porcelain

Height 28 cm

胎质坚硬。塑像光头垂耳，两颊深陷，长髯，喜笑颜开。身躯斜立，双手捧桃。寿星面部、手部及寿桃均施白釉，外衣、靴施褐色釉，内衣用绿色，飘带为黄色。

河北博物院藏

The hard and solid figurine has a shaven head with a pair of ears hanging down, sunken cheeks, and long beards. The figurine of the God of Longevity brims with smiles and stands slopingly with a peach in his hands. His cheeks, hands and the peach are glazed white, outer garment and boots brown, inner gown green, and ribbons yellow.

Preserved in Hebei Museum

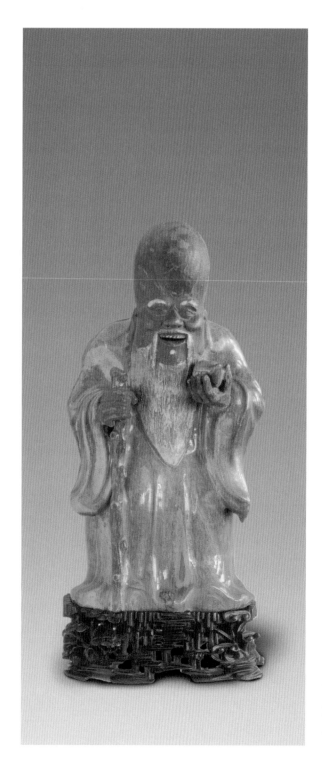

石湾窑翠毛釉寿星

清

瓷质

宽 20 厘米，高 38 厘米

Kingfisher Blue-glazed Figurine of God
of Longevity, Shiwan Kiln

Qing Dynasty

Porcelain

Width 20 cm/ Height 38 cm

石湾公仔名闻海内外。寿星白须白眉，头部
与手施以酱釉，右手拄杖，左手托桃，神态
活现，笑容可掬，衣褶简单而施釉厚重，造
型古拙，配以原装木座更是难能可贵，是石
湾公仔中的珍品。

高成藏

Shiwan stoneware is well known at home and
abroad. The figurine of the God of Longevity
with white beards and brows is radiant with
smiles. He is holding a walking stick in his right
hand and a peach in his left hand. His head and
hands are glazed dark reddish brown while his
gown with uncomplicated wrinkles is glazed
thickly. In spite of its unsophisticated shape,
it is even rare that the wooden stand below is
original. This figurine is a treasure trove among
them.

Collected by Gao Cheng

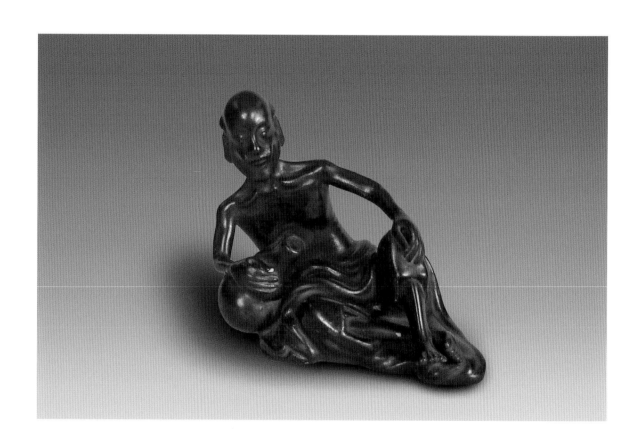

达摩瓷像

清

瓷质

宽 13.9 厘米，厚 9.2 厘米，通高 13.1 厘米

Porcelain Figurine of Bodhidharma

Qing Dynasty

Porcelain

Width 13.9 cm/ Thickness 9.2 cm/ Height 13.1 cm

人像形。该藏通身施黑色釉，为达摩神坐扶

葫芦的形象。工艺品。1954 年入藏，有残。

中华医学会 / 上海中医药大学医史博物馆

This work of art is the figurine of Bodhidharma,
who sits with a gourd between his right side
and right hand. The slightly damaged figurine
is glazed black all over. It was collected by
the museum in 1954.

Preserved in Chinese Medical Association/
Museum of Chinese Medicine, Shanghai
University of Traditional Chinese Medicine

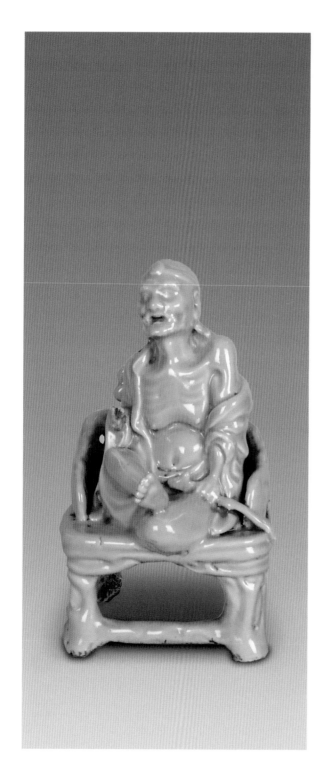

铁拐李像

清

瓷质

宽 10 厘米，厚 8 厘米，通高 17.6 厘米

Figurine of Li Tieguai

Qing Dynasty

Porcelain

Width 10 cm/ Thickness 8 cm/ Height 17.6 cm

人像形。该藏通身施绿灰釉，为铁拐李双
腿盘坐于藤椅上之像，左手持手杖。工艺
一般。工艺品。1958 年入藏，已残。

中华医学会 / 上海中医药大学医史博物馆

This work of art made with ordinary technique
is the figurine of Li Tieguai, one of the Eight
Immortals in Chinese legend. He sits cross-
legged on a vine chair with a stick in his left
hand. It was collected by the museum in 1958.
The figurine glazed greenish gray is broken.
Preserved in Chinese Medical Association/
Museum of Chinese Medicine, Shanghai
University of Traditional Chinese Medicine

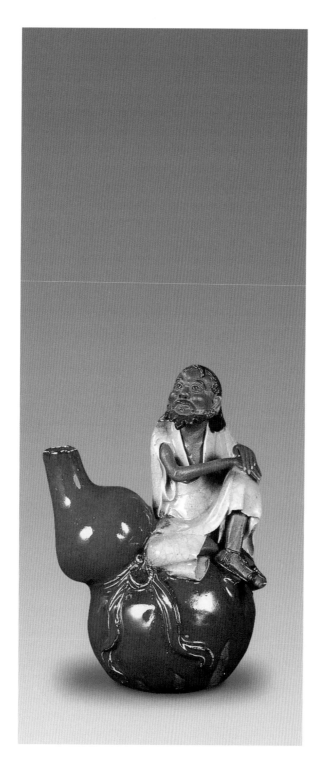

李铁拐瓷雕像

清

瓷质

底径 8 厘米，高 16 厘米

Porcelain Figurine of Li Tieguai

Qing Dynasty

Porcelain

Bottom Diameter 8 cm/ Height 16 cm

李铁拐，传说中的"八仙"之一，常在民间医治疾病。此像盘坐于葫芦上，双手置于腿上，脸上仰，面微笑，线条简练生动。

上海中医药博物馆藏

Li Tieguai, one of the Eight Immortals in Chinese legend, often treated illnesses of ordinary people. His figurine sits with crossed legs on a gourd and his hands on his leg. He looks upward, smiling. The lines are simple but lively.

Preserved in Shanghai Museum of Traditional Chinese Medicine

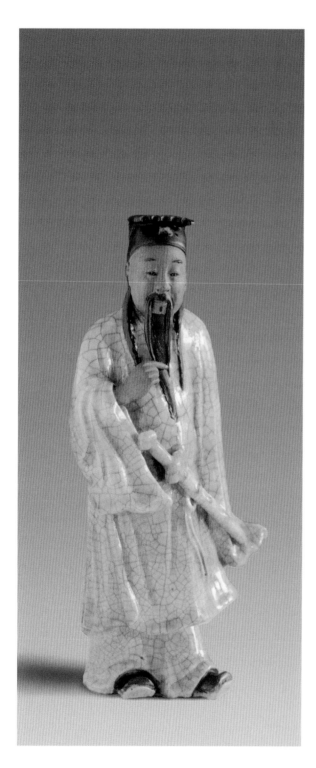

仿哥釉吕洞宾像

清

瓷质

高 27 厘米

Figurine of Lü Dongbin with Copied
Ge-style Glaze

Qing Dynasty

Porcelain

Height 27 cm

釉面开片。吕洞宾，传说中的"八仙"之一。钟吕内丹派代表人物，有"医神"之称。此立像慈眉善目，手缕胡须，腰佩宝剑，线条明快简练。

许荣坤藏

Lü Dongbin was one of the Eight Immortals in Chinese legend and the representative of Dan School. His standing figurine with a smiling face fondles its beard with its right hand and carries a sword around its waist. There are cracks on its surface. The lines are simple but lively.

Collected by Xu Rongkun

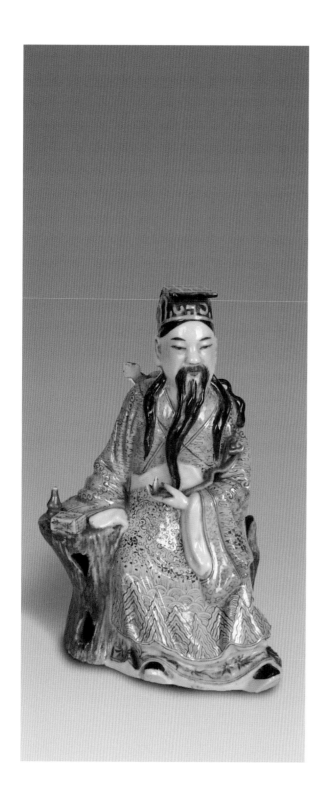

吕纯阳像

清

瓷质

宽 14.8 厘米，通高 22.3 厘米

Figurine of Lü Chunyang

Qing Dynasty

Porcelain

Width 14.8 cm/ Height 22.3 cm

人像形。该藏粉彩釉，为吕仙坐于石凳上，左手托一如意，右手边置本草书卷和葫芦瓶，背挎佩剑，造型生动美观。为工艺品。1954 年入藏，保存基本完好。

中华医学会 / 上海中医药大学医史博物馆

This work of art is the figurine of Lü Chunyang, also known as Lü Dongbin, one of the Eight Immortals of Chinese legend. He sits on a stone stool with a ruyi scepter in his left hand, a book on Chinese herbal medicine and a gourd-shaped bottle besides his right hand, and a sword on his back. The vivid and exquisite figurine is glazed famille rose palette. It was collected by the museum in 1954 and is basically in good condition.

Preserved in Chinese Medical Association/ Museum of Chinese Medicine, Shanghai University of Traditional Chinese Medicine

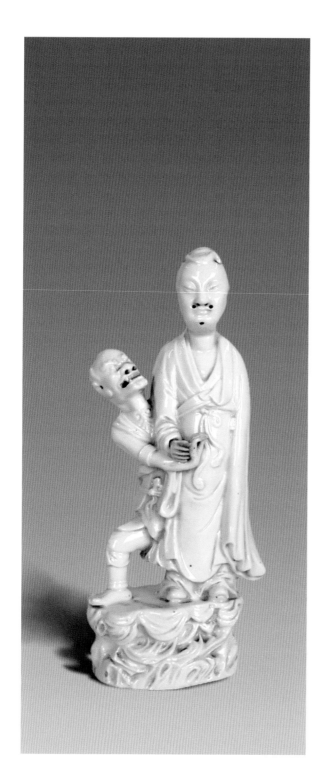

吕纯阳与柳树精瓷像

清

瓷质

宽 10.6 厘米，厚 8.7 厘米，通高 31 厘米

Porcelain Figurine of Lü Chunyang and Goblin of Willow

Qing Dynasty

Porcelain

Width 10.6 cm/ Thickness 8.7 cm/ Height 31 cm

人像形。该藏通身施白釉，为吕纯阳和柳树精双人弄法形象。工艺品。1954 年入藏，保存完好 。

中华医学会 / 上海中医药大学医史博物馆

The work of art is the figurine of Lü Chunyang, one of the Eight Immortals, and the goblin of willow, who are matching their magic powers. The figurine glazed white all over was collected by the museum in 1954 and is in good condition.

Preserved in Chinese Medical Association/ Museum of Chinese Medicine, Shanghai University of Traditional Chinese Medicine

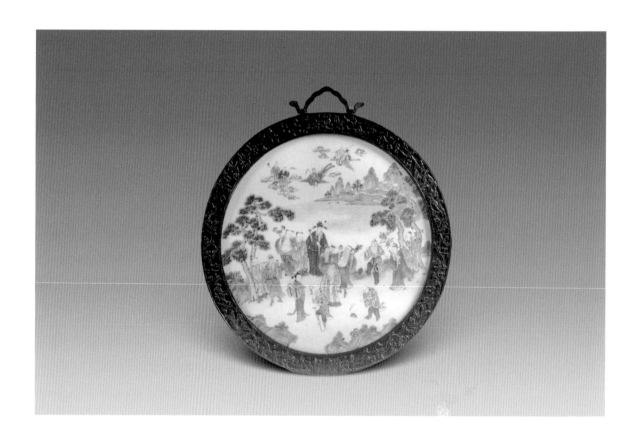

粉彩山水人物圆形瓷屏

清

瓷质

直径 43.6 厘米

Round Porcelain Screen Patterned with Landscape and Figures in Famille Rose Palette

Qing Dynasty

Porcelain

Diameter 43.6 cm

圆形瓷板。彩绘山水小景，一群仙人从远方来，或乘云，或骑鹤，或驾凤，下面群仙聚会，应为群仙祝寿的场面。神态各异，相互呼应，色彩鲜艳，是一幅精彩的山水人物瓷屏。

区子谦藏

The round porcelain screen is painted with landscape and figures: a group of immortals from the far distance are riding by clouds, on cranes or phoenixes for a party of numerous immortals, who seem to be extending good wishes on birthday. It is a wonderful scene in that everyone wears different facial expressions, the composition is well arranged, and the colors are bright.

Collected by Qu Ziqian

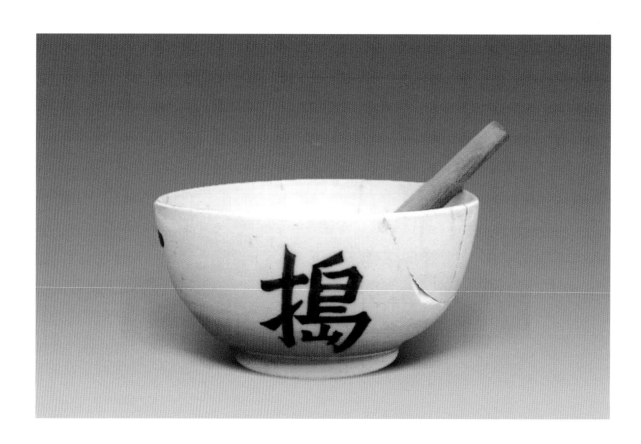

擂钵

清

瓷质

口径 22 厘米，高 12 厘米

Mortar and Pestle

Qing Dynasty

Porcelain

Mouth Diameter 22 cm/ Height 12 cm

外壁有蓝色釉书 7.5 厘米见方之"捣石研金"4 字。

似为炼丹用具。

广东中医药博物馆藏

The exterior wall of the mortar is inscribed with four blue-glazed words "Dao Shi Yan Jin" (pounding stones and grinding metals), each being 7.5 cm in square shape. This collection was apparently an alchemical tool.

Preserved in Guangdong Chinese Medicine Museum

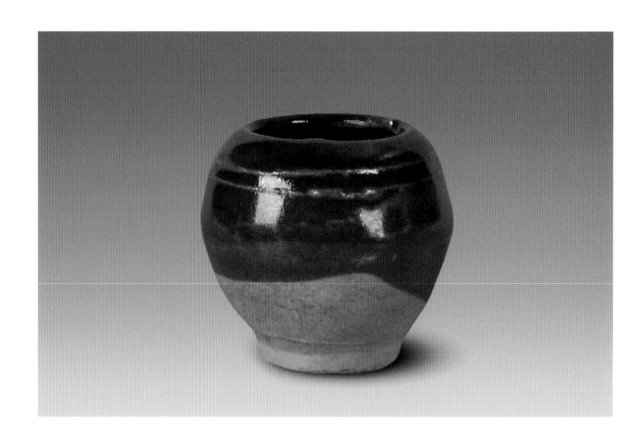

火罐

清

陶质

口径 2.9 厘米，腹径 4.4 厘米，底径 2.3 厘米，通高 4 厘米

Cupping Jar

Qing Dynasty

Pottery

Mouth Diameter 2.9 cm/ Belly Diameter 4.4 cm/ Bottom Diameter 2.3 cm/ Height 4 cm

罐形。该藏施酱色釉，下部和底无釉，旋纹，平底敛口，小巧玲珑，工艺一般。用于拔火罐。1962 年入藏，保存基本完好。

中华医学会 / 上海中医药大学医史博物馆

The delicate cupping jar made with ordinary technique is glazed dark reddish brown except for the lower part and the base. It has a contracted mouth, a flat base, and bowstring patterns around the body. The jar was collected by the museum in 1962 and is basically in good condition.

Preserved in Chinese Medical Association/ Museum of Chinese Medicine, Shanghai University of Traditional Chinese Medicine

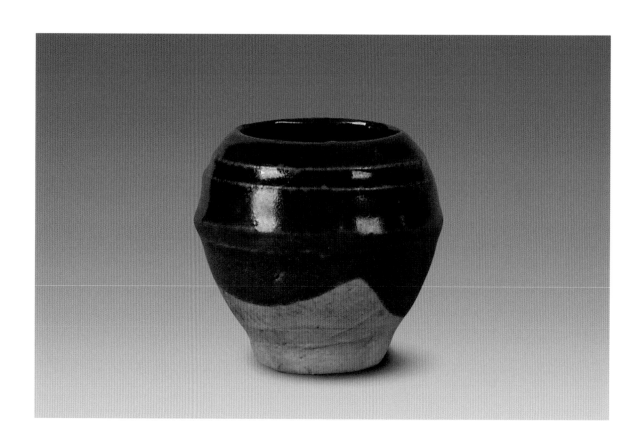

火罐

清

陶质

口径 2.9 厘米，腹径 4.4 厘米，底径 2.3 厘米，通高 4 厘米

Cupping Jar

Qing Dynasty

Pottery

Mouth Diameter 2.9 cm/ Belly Diameter 4.4 cm/ Bottom Diameter 2.3 cm/ Height 4 cm

罐形。该藏施酱色釉，下部和底无釉，旋纹，平底敛口，小巧玲珑工艺一般。用于拔火罐。1962 年入藏，保存基本完好。

中华医学会 / 上海中医药大学医史博物馆

The delicate cupping jar made with ordinary technique is glazed dark reddish brown except for the lower part and the base. It has a contracted mouth, a flat base, and bowstring patterns around the body. The jar was collected by the museum in 1962 and is basically in good condition.

Preserved in Chinese Medical Association/ Museum of Chinese Medicine, Shanghai University of Traditional Chinese Medicine

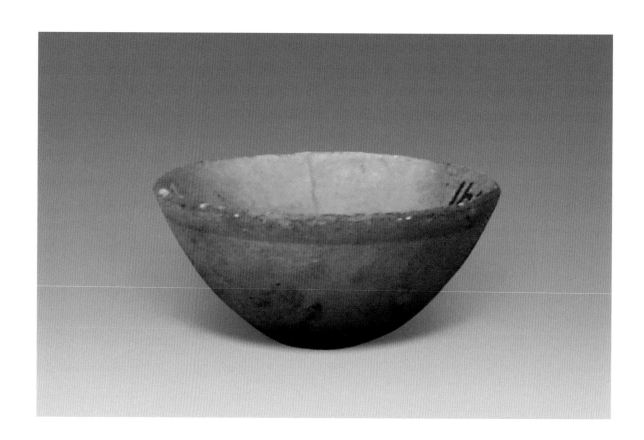

阳城罐

清

陶质

口径 7.2 厘米，通高 3.4 厘米

Yangcheng Earthen Bowl

Qing Dynasty

Pottery

Mouth Diameter 7.2 cm/ Height 3.4cm

棕黄陶制成。钵形。尖底敞口，工艺一般。为炼丹制药器具。1954 年入藏，保存基本完好。

中华医学会 / 上海中医药大学医史博物馆

The earthen bowl of ordinary technique is made of brownish yellow pottery. It has an everted mouth and a tapered body. It was used for making pills of immorality or for pharmacy. It was collected by the museum in 1954 and is basically in good condition.

Preserved in Chinese Medical Association/ Museum of Chinese Medicine, Shanghai University of Traditional Chinese Medicine

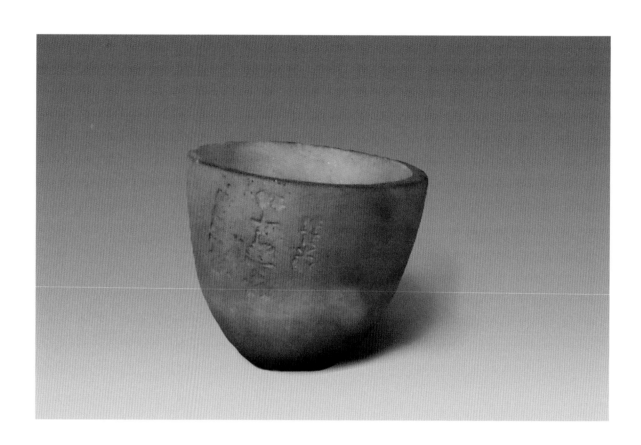

阳城罐

清

陶质

口径 9.7 厘米，通高 8 厘米

Yangcheng Earthen Bowl

Qing Dynasty

Pottery

Mouth Diameter 9.7 cm/ Height 8 cm

圆钵形。棕黄陶制成。尖底敞口，工艺一般，
表面有文字待考。为炼丹制药工具。1954 年
入藏，保存基本完好。

中华医学会 / 上海中医药大学医史博物馆

The round earthen bowl of ordinary technique is
made of brownish yellow pottery. It has an open
mouth and a tapered body with characters that
have yet to be verified. It was used for making
pills of immorality or for pharmacy. The bowl
was collected by the museum in 1954 and is
basically in good condition.

Preserved in Chinese Medical Association/
Museum of Chinese Medicine, Shanghai
University of Traditional Chinese Medicine

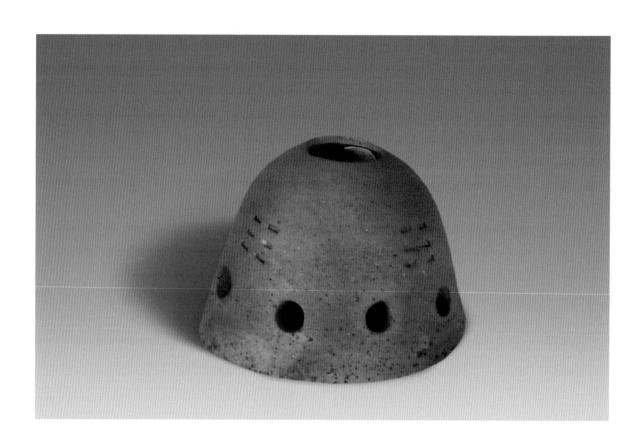

阳城罐

清

陶质

口径 12.3 厘米，通高 8 厘米

Yangcheng Earthen Bowl

Qing Dynasty

Pottery

Mouth Diameter 12.3 cm/ Height 8 cm

钵状。罐身有九个小孔，并浅刻八卦图案，是炼丹用具的一种。1954 年入藏。

中华医学会 / 上海中医药大学医史博物馆

The earthen bowl made of brownish yellow pottery was used for making pills of immorality. It has nine holes on its body and is incised shallowly with patterns of the Eight Diagrams in Chinese mythology. It was collected by the museum in 1954.

Preserved in Chinese Medical Association/ Museum of Chinese Medicine, Shanghai University of Traditional Chinese Medicine

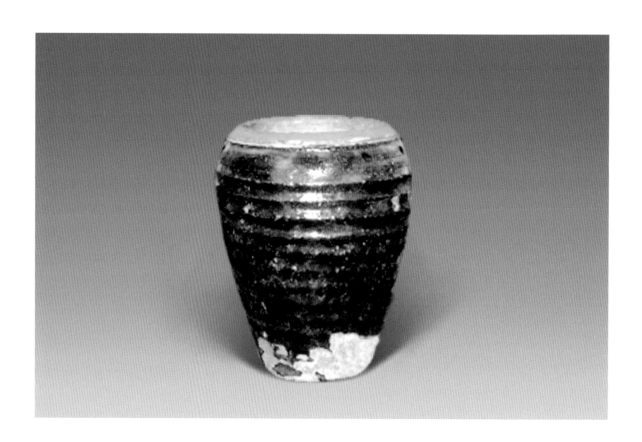

羊城罐

清

瓷质

口径 11 厘米，底径 7 厘米，通高 15 厘米，重 950 克

Yangcheng Earthen Jar

Qing Dynasty

Porcelain

Mouth Diameter 11 cm/ Bottom Diameter 7 cm/ Height 15 cm/ Weight 950 g

敞口，斜腹，平底，黑粗瓷，周身为筐纹。盛贮器。

完整无损。陕西省三原县征集。

陕西医史博物馆藏

The jar has an everted mouth, an inclined body, and a flat bottom. The coarse pottery body is glazed black and decorated with patterns of raised horizontal ridges. It was used for storage. The artifact was collected from Sanyuan County, Shaanxi Province, and is still in good condition.

Preserved in Shaanxi Museum of Medical History

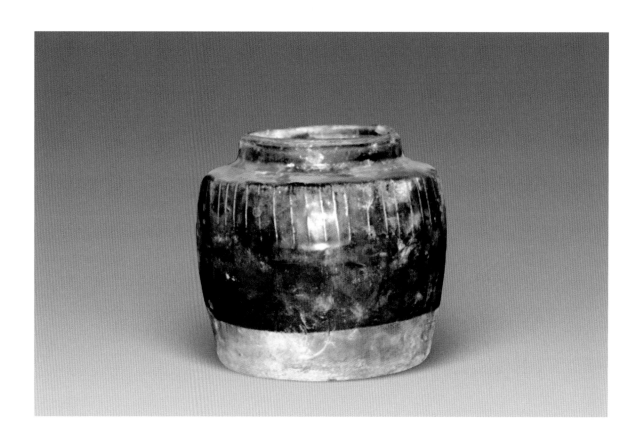

黑瓷罐

清

瓷质

口径 12.5 厘米，底径 17 厘米，通高 18 厘米，重 1700 克

Black Porcelain Jar

Qing Dynasty

Porcelain

Mouth Diameter 12.5 cm/ Bottom Diameter 17 cm/ Height 18 cm/ Weight 1,700 g

直口，直腹，平肩，上腹有一圈竖道，下腹有
一寸高白胎无釉。盛贮器。完整无损。

陕西医史博物馆藏

The jar has a vertical mouth, a vertical belly, and
a flat shoulder. The upper belly is decorated with
a circle of vertical lines and the lower belly has
a length of one-third decimeter unglazed white
pottery body. The jar used for storage is well
preserved.

Preserved in Shaanxi Museum of Medical History

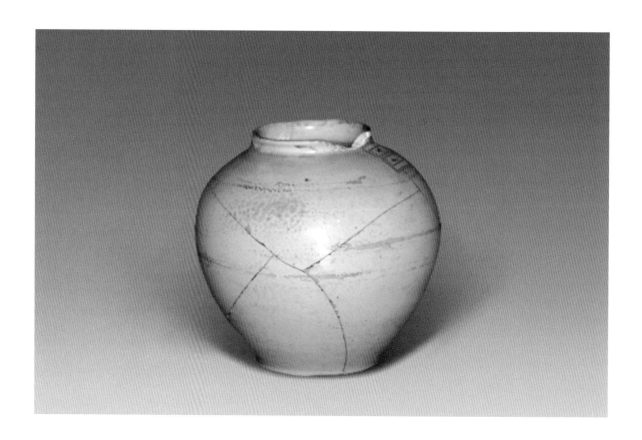

白釉瓷罐

清

瓷质

口径 8.5 厘米，底径 9 厘米，通高 16.5 厘米，重 1350 克

White-glazed Porcelain Jar

Qing Dynasty

Porcelain

Mouth diameter 8.5 cm/ Bottom Diameter 9 cm/ Height 16.5 cm/ Weight 1,350 g

圆唇，圆腹，平底。盛贮器。陕西省西安市东郊韩森寨征集。腹有修补。

陕西医史博物馆藏

The globular jar, which was used for storage, has a round mouth and a flat bottom. The belly has been repaired. It was collected from Hansenzhai, which lies on the eastern suburbs of Xi'an, Shaanxi Province.

Preserved in Shaanxi Museum of Medical History

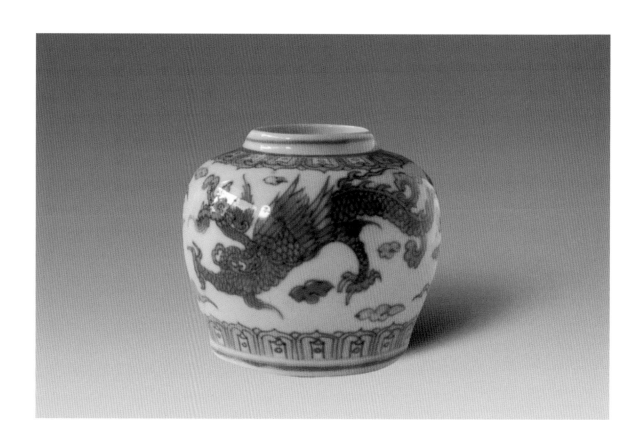

斗彩龙纹天字罐

清

瓷质

口径 4.7 厘米，底径 7.5 厘米，通高 8.5 厘米

Doucai Jar Painted with Dragons

Qing Dynasty

Porcelain

Mouth Diameter 4.7 cm/ Bottom Diameter 7.5 cm/ Height 8.5 cm

直口，短颈，丰肩至足渐收，矮圈足。颈中以青花画弦纹一周，颈和肩交界处以红彩画弦纹一道，肩部与近底部各彩绘变形覆仰莲纹带，腹间画双翼云龙相对。

谢志峰藏

The jar has a vertical mouth, a short neck, and a curved upper body which slightly tapers to the short ring foot. There is a circle of bowstring patterns in underglaze blue around the neck, with a red bowstring serving as the dividing line between the neck and the shoulder. The shoulder and the lower part are decorated with distorted upright lotus patterns in yellow and blue, with two dragons with a pair of wings facing each other in the middle.

Collected by Xie Zhifeng

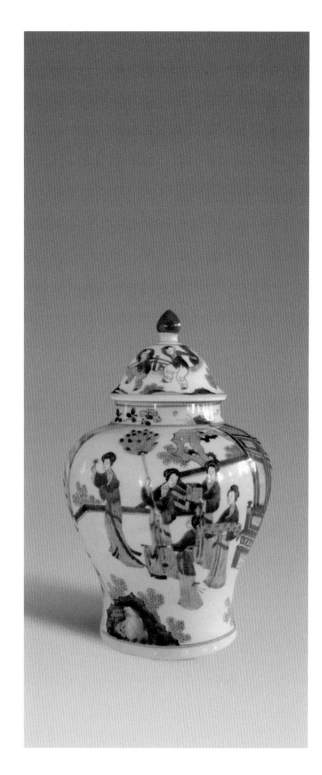

青花人物盖罐

清

瓷质

口径 10.3 厘米，腹围 66 厘米，足径 14.5 厘米，
通高 32 厘米

Lidded Jar Painted with Figures in Underglaze Blue

Qing Dynasty

Porcelain

Mouth Diameter 10.3 cm/ Belly Diameter 66 cm/
Bottom Diameter 14.5 cm/ Height 32 cm

罐有盖，宝珠钮。直口稍内收，短颈，丰肩
至足渐收，浅圈足。盖及罐身绘人物、风景
图案。白胎坚细，造型美观大方，釉色莹润
明亮，纹饰活泼自如。

李牧之藏

The jar has a lid with a pearl-shaped knob on
the top, a straight and slightly contracted mouth,
a short neck, and a bulged belly which tapers
to the short ring foot. The lid and the body are
painted with figures and landscape patterns. The
white pottery body is solid, fine and smooth; the
glaze is glossy; and the patterns are lively.
Collected by Li Muzhi

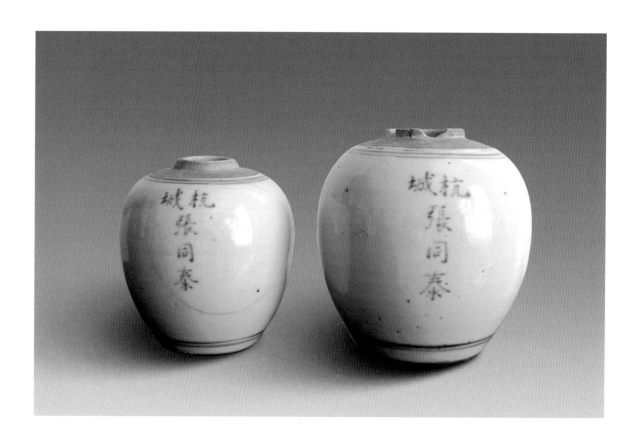

张同泰药罐

清

瓷质

左：腹径 12 厘米，高 11.5 厘米

右：腹径 13.5 厘米，高 13.5 厘米

Zhang Tongtai Medicine Bottle

Qing Dynasty

Porcelain

Left: Belly Diameter 12 cm/ Height 11.5 cm

Right: Belly Diameter 13.5 cm/ Height 13.5 cm

嘉庆十年（1805），张梅创建了张同泰药号。
同泰药号地处杭州同春坊孩儿巷口。

朱德明藏

The medicine brand name Zhang Tongtai was
created by Zhang Mei during the tenth year
of Jiaqing Reign (1805) of the Qing Dynasty.
The drug store named Tongtai is located at the
entrance of Lane Hai'er of Tongchun Road,
Hangzhou City.

Collected by Zhu Deming

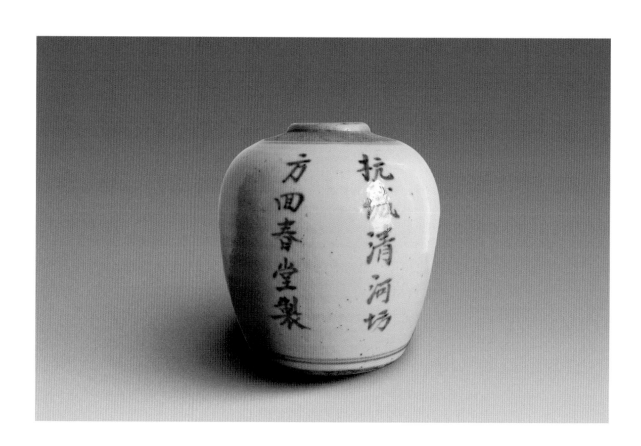

方回春堂药罐

清

瓷质

腹径 12.5 厘米，高 13 厘米

Fang Hui Chun Tang Medicine Bottle

Qing Dynasty

Porcelain

Belly Diameter 12.5 cm/ Height 13 cm

清顺治六年（1649），钱塘（今杭州）人
方清怡在望江门码头创办了国药号"方回春
堂"。

朱德明藏

The medicine brand name Fang Hui Chun
Tang was created by Fang Qingyi, a native of
Qiantang (the present Hangzhou City), at Wang
Jiangmen Dock during the sixth year of Shunzhi
Reign (1649) of the Qing Dynasty.
Collected by Zhu Deming

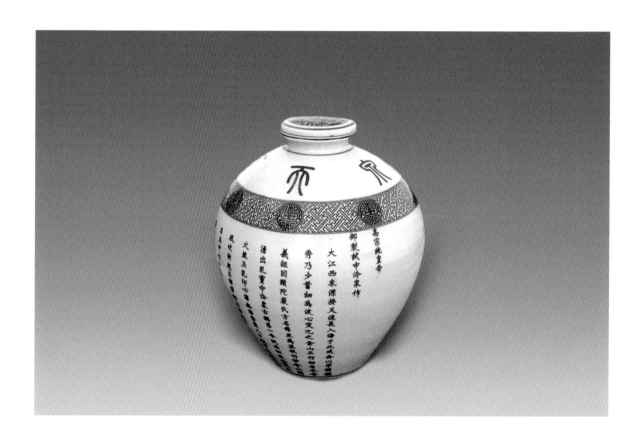

宫廷"天下第一泉"瓷坛

清

瓷质

腹径 35 厘米，通高 45 厘米

Palace Porcelain Jar Named "the Finest Spring Under Heaven"

Qing Dynasty

Porcelain

Belly Diameter 35 cm/ Height 45 cm

侈口，带盖，无钮，束颈，溜肩，鼓腹，平底，圆圈足，上有铭文"高宗纯皇帝""御制试中冷泉作"等。系清宫中之贮水容器。

广东中医药博物馆藏

The jar has a flared mouth, a knobless lid, a narrow neck, a sloping shoulder, a bulged belly, a flat bottom, and a ring foot. It is inscribed with words "Emperor Gao Zongchun" and words indicating the name of the imperial fine spring. The jar was used to store water in the imperial palace of the Qing Dynasty.

Preserved in Guangdong Chinese Medicine Museum

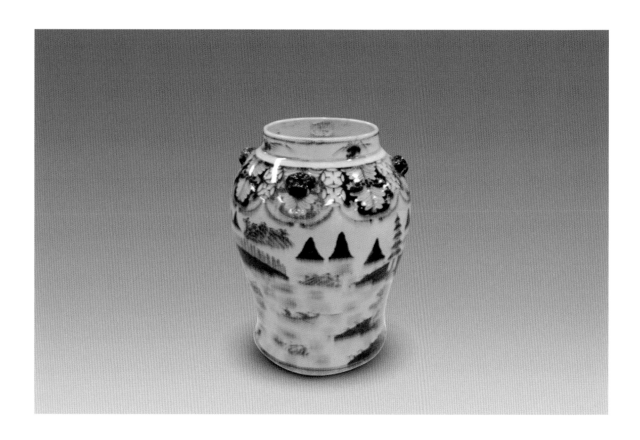

骨灰坛

清

瓷质

口径 22 厘米，底径 30 厘米，高 47 厘米

Cinerary Urn

Qing Dynasty

Porcelain

Mouth Diameter 22 cm/ Bottom Diameter 30 cm/ Height 47 cm

直口，肩微鼓，其下向内稍敛，至底部又微敞，平底，器身饰青花山水人物图案，肩部贴塑四个兽形钮。器形敦实浑厚，青花纹饰生动莹润。由成都博物馆调拨。

成都中医药大学中医药传统文化博物馆藏

The urn has a vertical mouth as well as a flat bottom and sides that slightly bulge to the shoulder, then taper a little and then evert to the bottom. There are four animal-shaped knobs on the shoulder and lively figures and landscape in underglaze blue on the exterior. The urn is sturdy, heavy and glossy. It was allocated from Chengdu Museum.

Preserved in Museum of Traditional Chinese Medicine Culture, Chengdu University of Traditional Chinese Medicine

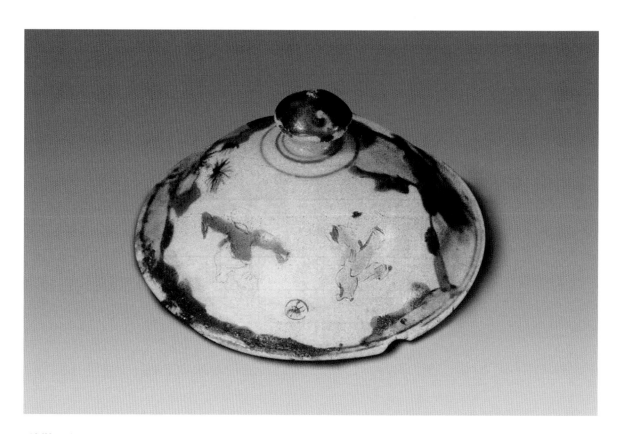

蹴鞠图五彩瓷坛盖

清

瓷质

口径 20 厘米，通高 15 厘米

Famille Verte Porcelain Jar-lid Painted with Children Playing Cuju Ball

Qing Dynasty

Porcelain

Mouth Diameter 20 cm/ Height 15 cm

盖为菌形钮，蹴鞠图绘于盖的外部。图中，
两童子正伸展双臂，抬腿踢足做蹴鞠状，中
间有一被踢起的球。画面生动活泼，颇具生
活气息。

中国体育博物馆藏

The lid with a mushroom-shaped knob is
painted with two children playing a cuju ball:
the children with arms stretched and legs lifted
are about to kick the ball, which is flying in the
air. The scene is full of vitality.

Preserved in China Sports Museum

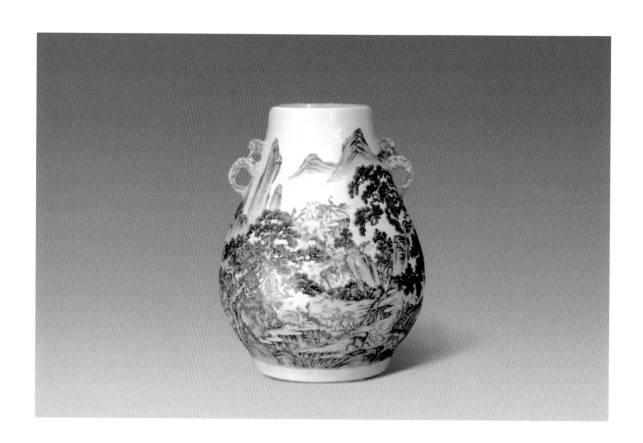

百鹿尊

清

瓷质

口径 17 厘米，通高 42 厘米

Zun Vessel Painted with Numerous White Deer

Qing Dynasty

Porcelain

Mouth Diameter 17 cm/ Height 42 cm

口微敞，口以下渐放，腹下部丰满，圈足，肩部贴螭形双耳，形似牛头，故亦称"牛头尊"。通体施白釉，腹部粉彩彩绘百鹿活跃于山林之中。

山西博物院藏

The zun vessel, which has a slightly everted mouth, stretching sides, bulged belly, a ring foot, and a pair of hornless dragon-shaped ears on the shoulder, is shaped like a bull's head; thus it is called "Niutou Zun" (bull head-shaped zun vessel). The vessel is coated with white glaze all over and painted with numerous deer in famille rose amid trees and hills.

Preserved in Shanxi Museum

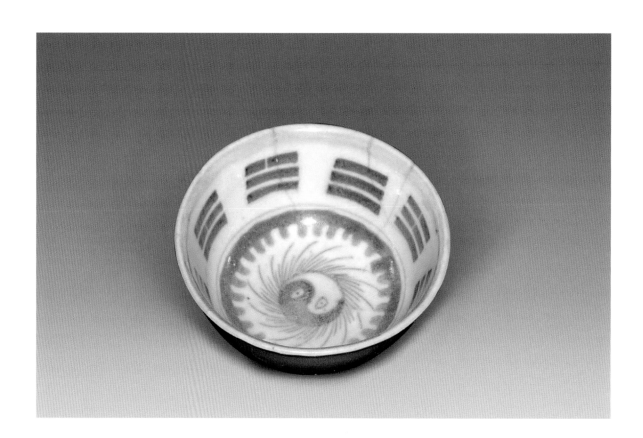

八卦瓷瓶

清

瓷质

口径 9.5 厘米，底径 4.3 厘米，通高 5 厘米，重 100 克

Porcelain Bowl Painted with the Eight Diagrams in Chinese Mythology

Qing Dynasty

Porcelain

Mouth Diameter 9.5 cm/ Bottom Diameter 4.3 cm/ Height 5 cm/ Weight 100 g

敞口，直斜腹，拱壁足，碗内有太极八卦图，外豆绿色。生活用器。陕西省澄城县征集。有裂印。

陕西医史博物馆藏

The bowl has a flared mouth, a straight and sloping belly, and an arched foot. It is painted with the Eight Diagrams in Chinese mythology on the interior and glazed bean green on the exterior. This household utensil with cracks was collected from Chengcheng County, Shaanxi Province.

Preserved in Shaanxi Museum of Medical History

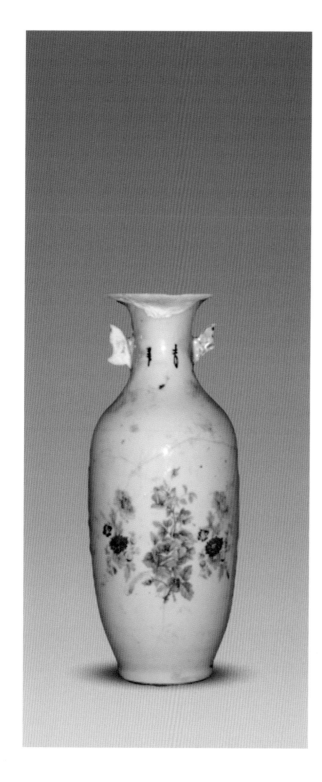

双耳瓷瓶

清

瓷质

口径 9 厘米，底径 7 厘米，通高 26.5 厘米，重 800 克

Porcelain Bottle with Double Ears

Qing Dynasty

Porcelain

Mouth Diameter 9 cm/ Bottom Diameter 7 cm/ Height 26.5 cm/ Weight 800 g

喇叭口，颈部有双耳，直腹，圈足，白瓷上施小红花，并题有诗词。盛贮器。口沿及一耳有修补。

陕西医史博物馆藏

The vase has a trumpet-shaped mouth, a pair of ears on the neck, a vertical belly, and a ring foot. The white-glazed body is decorated with tiny red flowers and a poem. The mouth rim and one ear have been repaired. The bottle was used for storage.

Preserved in Shaanxi Museum of Medical History

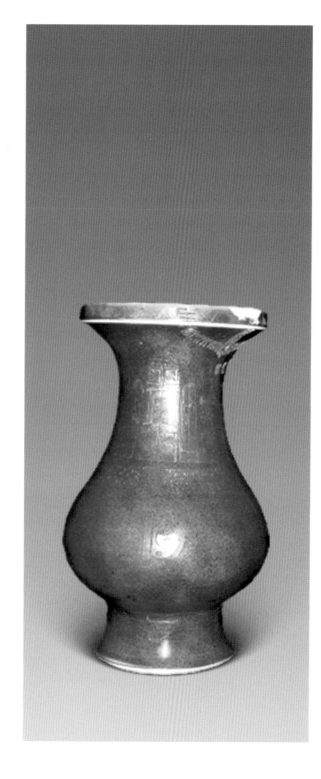

兰釉描金插瓶

清

瓷质

口径 20 厘米，底径 15.5 厘米，通高 36.5 厘米，重 4400 克

Blue-glazed Vase with Gold-outlined Patterns

Qing Dynasty

Porcelain

Mouth Diameter 20 cm/ Bottom Diameter 15.5 cm/ Height 36.5 cm/ Weight 4,400 g

盘口，长颈，鼓腹，喇叭底，圈足，描金兰釉。
艺术品。口有修补。

陕西医史博物馆藏

The vase has an erected mouth, a long neck, a bulged belly, a trumpet-shaped bottom, and a ring foot. It has patterns outlined in gold against the blue glaze on the exterior. The mouth of the work of art has been repaired.

Preserved in Shaanxi Museum of Medical History

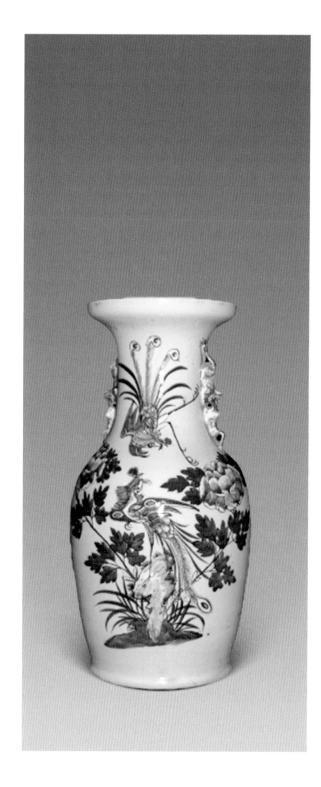

瓷插瓶

清

瓷质

口径 18 厘米，底径 17.5 厘米，通高 43 厘米，
重 4400 克

Porcelain Vase

Qing Dynasty

Porcelain

Mouth Diameter 18 cm/ Bottom Diameter 17.5 cm/
Height 43 cm/ Weight 4,400 g

盘口，长颈，圆肩，斜腹，圈足，四狮兽耳豆绿色，

双凤牡丹图。艺术品。陕西省鄠邑区谢家店征集。

完整无损。

陕西医史博物馆藏

The bean green-glazed vase has an erected mouth, a
long neck, a round shoulder, an inclined belly, a ring
foot, and a pair of ears each shaped like two opposing
lions. It is painted with a couple of phoenixes
amid peonies. The work of art was collected from
Xiejiadian of Huyi District, Shaanxi Province, and is
well preserved.

Preserved in Shaanxi Museum of Medical History

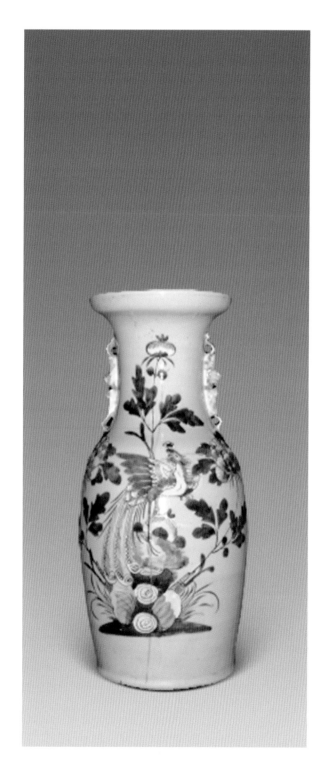

瓷插瓶

清

瓷质

口径 17 厘米，底径 17 厘米，通高 44 厘米，重 3600 克

Porcelain Vase

Qing Dynasty

Porcelain

Mouth Diameter 17 cm/ Bottom Diameter 17 cm/ Height 44 cm/ Weight 3,600 g

盘口，长颈，溜肩，斜腹，圈足，四狮兽耳，
豆绿色，凤凰牡丹图。艺术品。陕西省鄠邑区
谢家店中药店征集。完整无损。

陕西医史博物馆藏

The bean green-glazed vase has an erected mouth,
a long neck, an inclined belly, a ring foot, and a
pair of ears each shaped like two opposing lions.
It is painted with a couple of phoenixes amid
peonies. The work of art was collected from a
traditional Chinese medicine store in Xiejiadian
of Huyi District, Shaanxi Province, and is well
preserved.

Preserved in Shaanxi Museum of Medical History

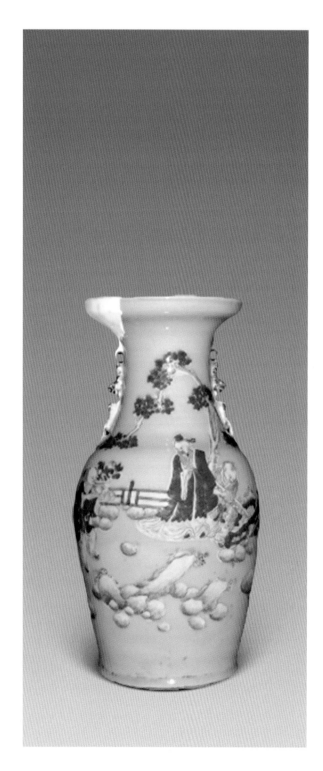

瓷插瓶

清

瓷质

口径 18 厘米，底径 17 厘米，通高 42 厘米，重 3400 克

Porcelain Vase

Qing Dynasty

Porcelain

Mouth Diameter 18 cm/ Bottom Diameter 17 cm/ Height 42 cm/ Weight 3,400 g

盘口，长颈，圆肩，斜腹，圈足，四狮兽耳豆绿色，

古树三人图。艺术品。陕西省汉中市公兴大药

店征集。口沿有修补。

陕西医史博物馆藏

The bean green-glazed vase has an erected mouth,
a long neck, a round shoulder, an inclined belly, a
ring foot, and a pair of ears each shaped like two
opposing lions. It is painted with three figures
under an ancient tree. The mouth rim of the work
of art has been repaired. The vase was collected
from Gong Xing Pharmacy in Hanzhong City,
Shaanxi Province.

Preserved in Shaanxi Museum of Medical History

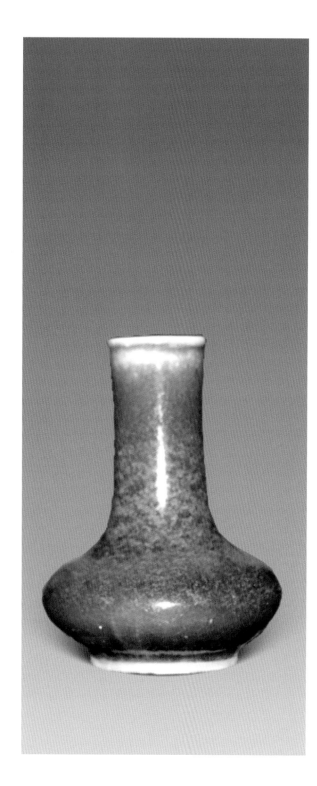

钧瓷插瓶

清

瓷质

口径 4.5 厘米，底径 7 厘米，通高 15 厘米，重 650 克

Jun-style Porcelain Vase

Qing Dynasty

Porcelain

Mouth Diameter 4.5 cm/ Bottom Diameter 7 cm/ Height 15 cm/ Weight 650 g

瓶为直口，长颈，鼓腹，圈足钧瓷带一底座。
生活用器。陕西省西安市征集。完整无损。

陕西医史博物馆藏

The Jun-style vase has a vertical mouth, a long
neck, a bulged belly, and a ring foot. The utensil
for daily use was collected from Xi'an, Shaanxi
Province, and is well preserved.

Preserved in Shaanxi Museum of Medical History

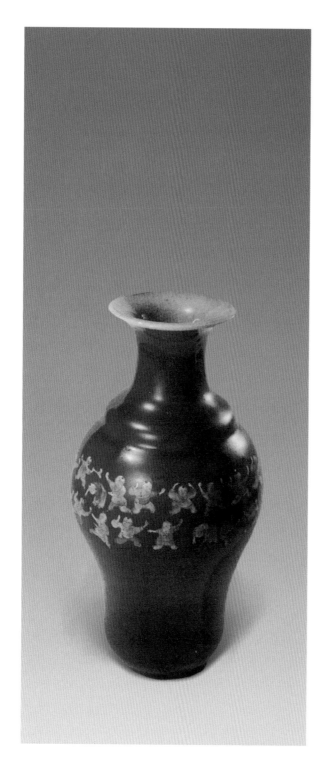

拳术演练纹红釉瓷瓶

清

瓷质

通高 40 厘米

Red-glazed Porcelain Vase Painted with Chinese Boxing Exercises Scene

Qing Dynasty

Porcelain

Height 40 cm

瓶为长颈，侈口，深腹，平底。拳术纹饰于腹部，一群习武者正在演练拳术套路，其中既有单人的演练，也有双人的对练，画面生动形象。

中国体育博物馆藏

The vase has a flared mouth, a long neck, a deep belly, and a flat bottom. The belly is painted with a scene of a group of figures doing Chinese boxing exercises, some of whom are practicing by themselves and some in pairs. The painting is full of vitality.

Preserved in China Sports Museum

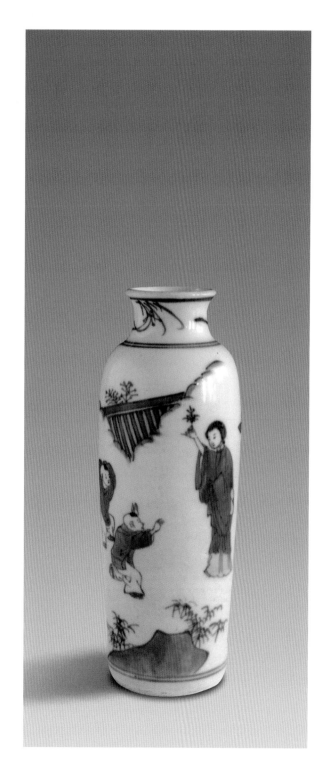

青花人物芭蕉纹筒子瓶

清

瓷质

口径 4.6 厘米，通高 20 厘米

Blue-and-white Tube-shaped Vase Painted with Figures and Plantains

Qing Dynasty

Porcelain

Mouth Diameter 4.6 cm/ Height 20 cm

瓶口稍外撇，短颈，溜肩，直身往下稍收成筒子形，平底。口沿画弦纹一道，绘垂兰数株，近颈处以及近足处各画双弦纹一道。腹间绘一手拈花草逗引孩童嬉戏的仕女及芭蕉竹石。胎体坚致厚重，洁白细润，器型古拙，青花淡雅，稍泛灰色，尚有晚明遗风。

高成藏

The vase has a slightly everted mouth, a short neck, a sloping shoulder, and a tube-shaped body that slightly tapers to the flat base. There are a bowstring around the mouth rim, several drooping orchids around the neck, and double bowstrings near both the shoulder and the foot. The belly is decorated with a lady with a flower in her hand tantalizing some children amid plantains, bamboos and stones. The characteristics of vases in the late Ming Dynasty can still be seen from the vase: the pottery body is hard, heavy and thick; the white porcelain is pure and glossy; the shape is unsophisticated; and the blue-and-white painting is elegant and slightly grayish.

Collected by Gao Cheng

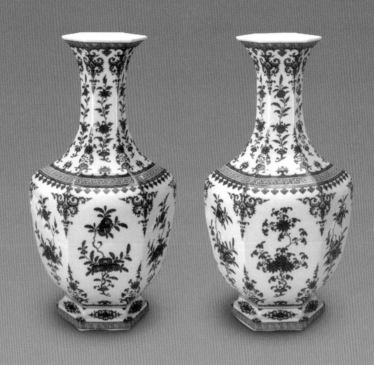

乾隆青花折枝花果纹六角瓶

清

瓷质

口径 18 厘米，通高 66 厘米

Blue-and-white Hexagonal Vases Patterned with Plucked Flowers and Fruits, Qianlong Reign

Qing Dynasty

Porcelain

Mouth Diameter 18 cm/ Height 66 cm

瓶为传世品。瓶通体作六方形，敞口，细高颈，折肩，深腹，外撇圈足，胎质洁白细腻，釉质莹润。通体绘鲜艳的青花图案，层次分明。口下、肩、圈足均绘回纹。颈部绘如意纹和各不相同的折枝花纹。腹部每面绘一组不同的折枝花果图案，有灵芝、寿桃等纹饰，并以如意花草作转角装饰，青花色泽雅致，纹饰丰富，器型硕大，是乾隆官窑精品。

扬州博物馆藏

The pair of vases have been handed down for generations. The hexagonal vases have everted mouths, long and narrow necks, sloping shoulders, deep bellies, and everted feet. The pottery body is white, pure and fine, and the glaze is glossy. There are bright blue-and-white patterns all over those vases; fret motifs close to the mouth rims, on the shoulders and feet; Ruyi motifs and various plucked flower motifs on the necks; plucked flower and fruit (including ganoderma and peaches) motifs which are different from each other on the sides; and Ruyi flowers and plants on the turning sides. The pair of huge vases with elegant underglaze blue glaze and rich adornment is one of the best among those made in governmental kilns during Qianlong Reign of the Qing Dynasty.

Preserved in Yangzhou Museum

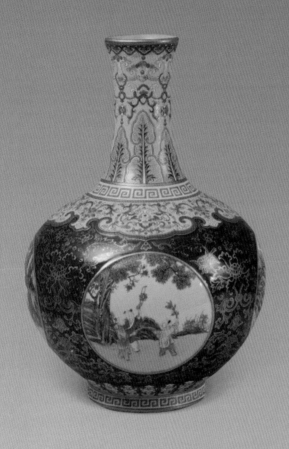

霁蓝釉粉彩婴戏纹天球瓶

清

瓷质

口径 8 厘米，足径 12 厘米，通高 34 厘米

Deep Blue-glazed Spherical Vase Painted with
Playing Children in Famille Rose Palette Enamel

Qing Dynasty

Porcelain

Mouth Diameter 8 cm/ Foot Diameter 12 cm/ Height 34 cm

器作天球瓶，喇叭形口，高颈，圆腹，圈足。腹部圆形开光内，月白色地，施粉彩绘顽童戏耍，以山石、松、梅为背景。开光之外，霁蓝釉地，施金彩绘缠枝莲花，画面开阔清新，粉彩淡雅柔丽，犹如国画作品，给人以舒适之感。底有红彩楷书"大清乾隆年制"款。乾隆帝赐予岱庙作祭。

泰安市博物馆藏

The spherical vase has a flared mouth, a long neck, a bulged belly, and a ring foot. On the exterior there is a bluish white roundel enclosing some naughty children playing and rockeries, pines and plum trees as the background. The children are painted with famille rose palette enamel. Outside the roundel there is a lotus scroll depicted with gold and some other patterns. The decorations enclosed by the roundels are just like traditional Chinese paintings. The paintings with wide views and elegant famille rose palette enamel are refreshing and comforting. The bottom of the vase is inscribed with red-glazed Chinese words "Da Qing Qian Long Nian Zhi" (made during Qianlong Reign of the Qing Dynasty) in regular script. The vase was bestowed by Emperor Qianlong on the Dai Temple as a sacrificial offering.

Preserved in Tai'an Museum

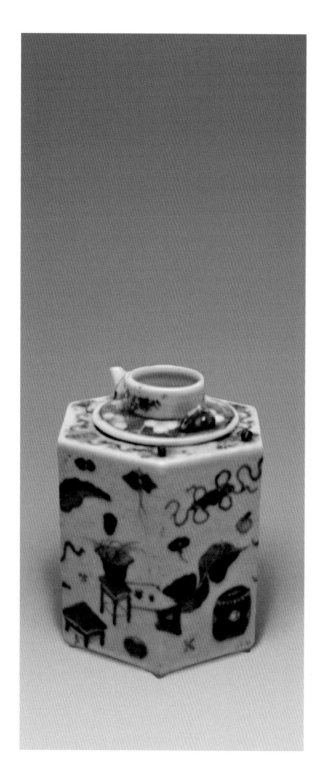

温酒器

清

瓷质

通高 7 厘米

Wine Warmer

Qing Dynasty

Porcelain

Height 7 cm

六角形。器身成柱状，四足，器物四周饰青花花草纹，中间的壶内盛酒，由内外层之间的热水烫热，不致伤胃，由民间征集。

成都中医药大学中医药传统文化博物馆藏

The hexagonal vessel, which has a columnar body and four feet, is painted with blue-and-white flowers, plants and other motifs. It has two layers of sides, between which boiled water could warm wine in the inner vessel, so as not to hurt the stomach. The artifact was collected from a private owner.

Preserved in Museum of Traditional Chinese Medicine Culture, Chengdu University of Traditional Chinese Medicine

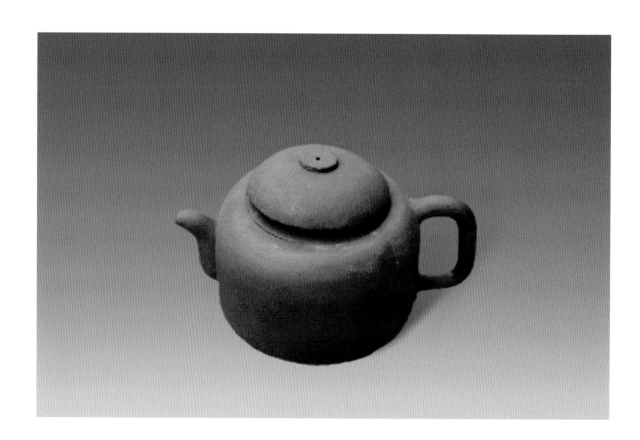

紫砂暖壶

清

陶质

外口径 6.58 厘米，腹径 11.6 厘米，壶深 6.6 厘米，通高 10.5 厘米，重 442 克

Zisha Thermos Pot

Qing Dynasty

Pottery

Mouth Outer Diameter 6.58 cm/ Belly Diameter 11.6 cm/ Depth 6.6 cm/ Height 10.5 cm/ Weight 442 g

形似茶壶，近方形耳，腹鼓而扁，平底，短流，用于取暖。

广东中医药博物馆藏

The vessel, which looks like a teapot, has a nearly square ear, a bulged and short belly, a flat bottom, and a short spout. It was used to keep warm.

Preserved in Guangdong Chinese Medicine Museum

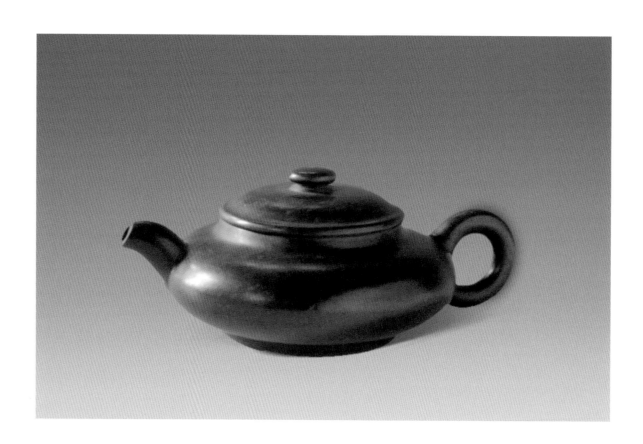

宜兴紫砂扁壶

清

紫砂

通高 10 厘米

Yixing Clay Flat Pot

Qing Dynasty

Zisha Pottery

Height 10 cm

壶身扁矮折腰，执手为环形，壶嘴短小，壶盖入口吻合无隙，整体造型圆浑可喜，沙质细腻，底部印"大亨"阳文楷书瓜子印。

杜灿佳藏

The pot has a depressed body, a ringlike handle, a short and tiny spout, a lid that fits in the body seamlessly, and a relief inscription "Da Heng" in regular script on the bottom. The pot made of fine clay is round and smooth.

Collected by Du Canjia

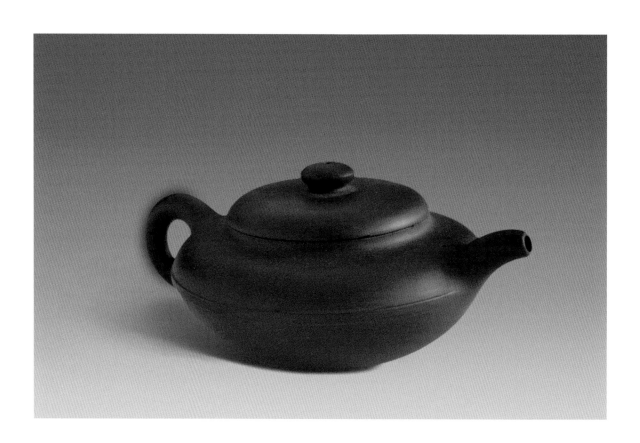

宜兴窑"大彬"款紫砂壶

清

紫砂

通高 13 厘米

Yixing Clay Teapot Inscribed with "Da Bin"

Qing Dynasty

Zisha Pottery

Height 13 cm

壶呈扁圆腹，直口，矮圈足。腹间装圆筒形流稍弯。与流相对处为圆条形半环柄，盖稍鼓，扁圆钮，圈足内刻行草"头影分光翠色浮大彬"铭款。褐紫砂胎，胎质坚密。器型温文尔雅，颇为优美。

高丰藏

The teapot has a depressed and round belly, a vertical mouth, and a short ring foot. There are a cylindrical spout slightly curved on the belly, a semicircular handle opposite the spout, a slightly bulged lid with an oblate knob at the center, and a nine-word inscription in running script on the ring foot. The terra-cotta clay is solid and thick, and the model is refined, gentle and elegant.

Collected by Gao Feng

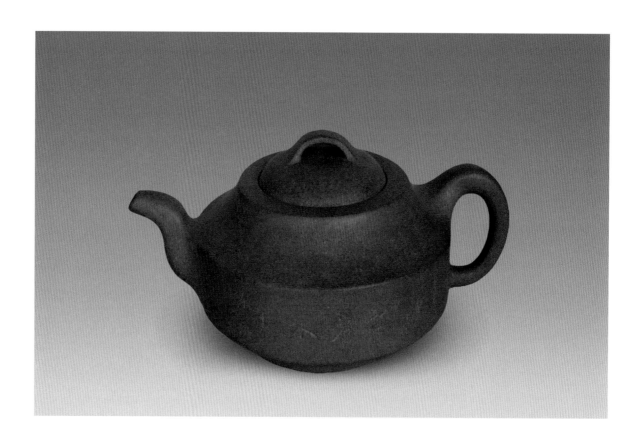

紫砂壶

清

紫砂陶

直径 12.25 厘米，宽 17.8 厘米，通高 7.7 厘米

Zisha Teapot

Qing Dynasty

Zisha Pottery

Diameter 12.25 cm/ Width 17.8 cm/ Height 7.7 cm

壶形。该藏由紫砂陶制成，平底，一端设桥状耳，一端为壶嘴，上配壶盖亦桥状钮。底和盖内均有款识（待考），壶身浅刻"龙芽初试碧水甘　东溪作于古阳钦"字样。为茶具。1957 年入藏。保存基本完好。

中华医学会 / 上海中医药大学医史博物馆

The teapot is made of Zisha or purple sand. It has a flat base, a bridge-shaped handle, a spout, a lid with a bridge-shaped handle on the top, inscriptions (unverified) on both the bottom and the interior of the lid, and Chinese characters shallowly incised on the body. The teapot was collected by the museum in 1957 and is basically by good condition.

Preserved in Chinese Medical Association/ Museum of Chinese Medicine, Shanghai University of Traditional Chinese Medicine

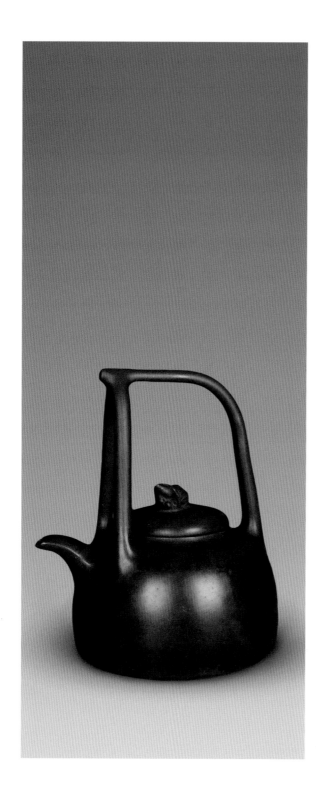

紫砂壶

清

紫砂

腹径 12.45 厘米，宽 14.3 厘米，通高 16.6 厘米

Zisha Teapot

Qing Dynasty

Zisha Pottery

Diameter 12.45 cm/ Width 14.3 cm/ Height 16.6 cm

茶壶形。该藏紫砂制成，表面光滑，圈足平底高提梁，提梁上有"赦记"款识，壶盖置卷叶钮，小壶嘴略弯，做工精细，造型美观。为茶具。1956 年入藏，保存基本完好。

中华医学会 / 上海中医药大学医史博物馆

The teapot made of Zisha or purple sand is smooth, exquisite and delicate. It has a ring foot, a flat bottom, a long handle inscribed with "She Ji" indicating the surname of the owner, a lid with a knob shaped like a curved leaf on the center, and a slightly bent tiny spout. The teapot was collected by the museum in 1956 and is basically in good condition.

Preserved in Chinese Medical Association/ Museum of Chinese Medicine, Shanghai University of Traditional Chinese Medicine

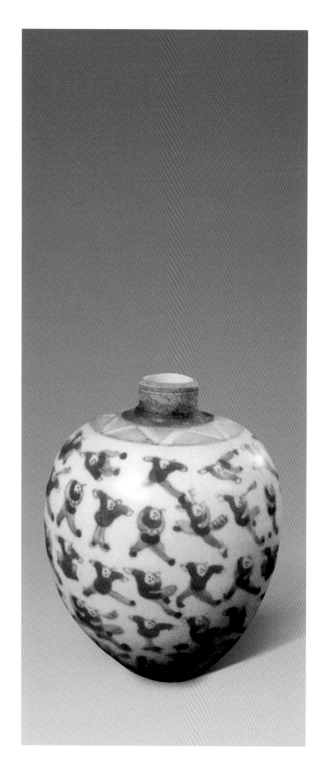

拳术演练纹青花瓷壶

清

瓷质

口径 5 厘米，腹径 13 厘米，通高 25 厘米

Blue-and-white Porcelain Jar Painted with Chinese Boxing Exercises

Qing Dynasty

Porcelain

Mouth Diameter 5 cm/ Belly Diameter 13 cm/

Height 25 cm

壶为小口，鼓腹，平底。拳术演练纹饰于壶的整个腹部，由上至下共分为四列，描绘了所演练拳术的一系列连贯动作。说明当时武术中拳术的套路已甚为丰富。

中国体育博物馆藏

The jar has a small mouth, a bulged belly, and a flat bottom. Its entire body is painted with a series of successive Chinese boxing movements arranged in four rows, which indicates that the set patterns of Chinese boxing were rich at that time.

Preserved in China Sports Museum

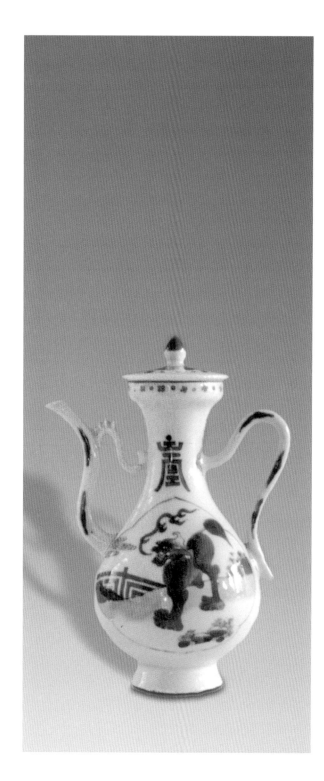

青花狮子纹执壶

清

瓷质

口径 5.8 厘米，底径 5.8 厘米，通高 21 厘米

Blue-and-white Kettle Painted with Unicorn

Qing Dynasty

Porcelain

Mouth Diameter 5.8 cm/ Bottom Diameter 5.8 cm/ Height 21 cm

盘口，长颈，溜肩，鼓腹，圈足外撇，有盖。肩部装圆筒弯曲形长流，以 S 形条接于流和颈间，与流相对处外装扁条形执。口沿以小十字和圆点纹相间绕沿一周，颈部书寿字，腹两边为桃形开光，内绘独角兽和云纹，简洁粗放。施白釉匀净莹亮，器形端正，线条优美，堪称民窑的佳作。

刘坚藏

The kettle has an erected mouth, a long neck, a sloping shoulder, a bulged belly, a flared ring foot, and a lid. There is a curved cylindrical spout on the belly, an S-shaped strip collecting the spout with the neck, and a strip handle on the opposite side. There are tiny cross motifs and dots arranged alternately around the rim, a word "Shou" (longevity) on the neck, two peach-shaped panels on the opposite sides on the belly, and an unicorn and cloud motifs on each panel. With glossy and even white glaze, neat shape and elegant lines, the kettle can be regarded as an excellent one among those made in non-governmental kilns.

Collected by Liu Jian

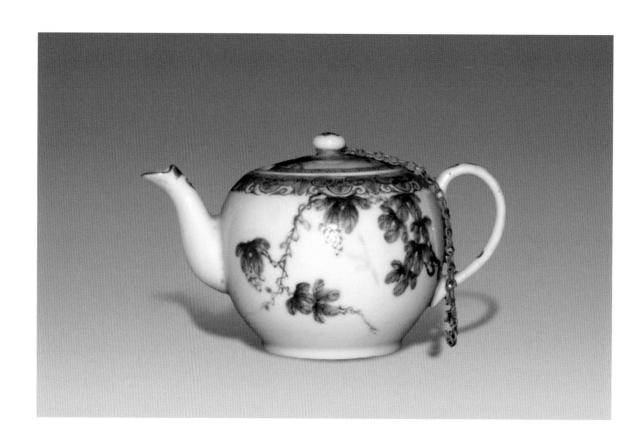

茶壶

清

瓷质

口径 7.5 厘米，底径 7 厘米，通高 11 厘米，重 350 克

Teapot

Qing Dynasty

Porcelain

Mouth Diameter 7.5 cm/ Bottom Diameter 7 cm/ Height 11 cm/ Weight 350 g

子母口，圆腹，圈足，底有"乾隆年制"字把和
盖之间带银链。茶具，生活用器具。陕西中医药
大学袁立新老师家传捐赠。完整无损。

陕西医史博物馆藏

The teapot has a snap-lid, a round belly, and a ring
foot. The bottom is inscribed with Chinese words
"Qian Long Nian Zhi" (made during Qianlong
Reign). A silver chain connects the handle with
the lid. The teapot, which was an article for daily
use, is well preserved. The handed-down artifact
was donated by Yuan Lixin, a teacher of Shaanxi
College of Traditional Chinese Medicine.
Preserved in Shaanxi Museum of Medical History

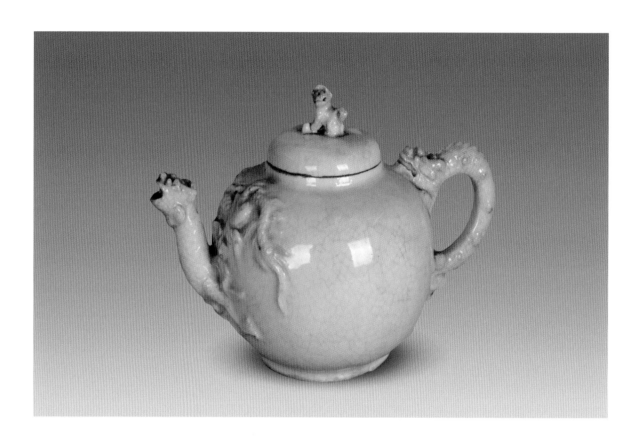

茶壶

清

瓷质

宽 16.6 厘米，通高 10.4 厘米

Teapot

Qing Dynasty

Porcelain

Width 16.6 cm/ Height 10.4 cm

茶壶形。乳白釉，小开片，龙桥耳，龙舌嘴，上盖配兽钮，圈足平底，工艺较好。为茶具。1957 年入藏，保存基本完好。

中华医学会 / 上海中医药大学医史博物馆

The teapot, which is coated with milky glaze with small crackles, has a dragon-shaped handle, a dragon tongue-shaped spout, an animal-shaped knob, a ring foot and a flat bottom The fine vessel was collected by the museum in 1957 and is basically well preserved.

Preserved in Chinese Medical Association/ Museum of Chinese Medicine, Shanghai University of Traditional Chinese Medicine

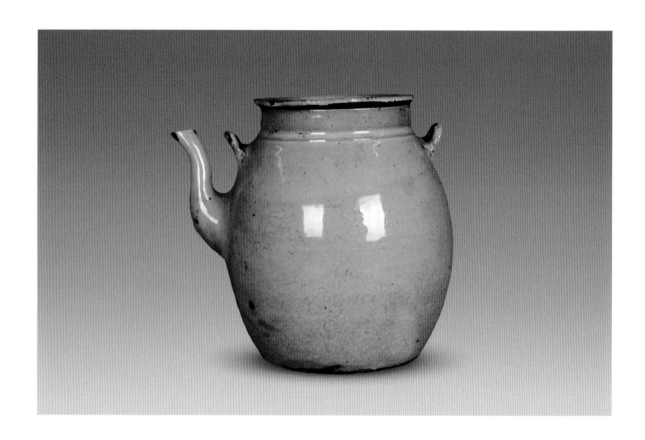

茶壶

清

瓷质

宽 16.4 厘米，通高 15 厘米

Teapot

Qing Dynasty

Porcelain

Width 16.4 cm/ Height 15 cm

壶形。该藏通身施青灰釉，釉下旋纹明显，平底敞口，有盖无提梁，嘴略弯曲，肩部有两系四孔，底无款，壶内面露土褐色胎，工艺一般。为茶具。1955 年入藏，保存基本完好。

中华医学会 / 上海中医药大学医史博物馆

The teapot, which has clear bowstring patterns under the bluish gray glaze but no inscription on the bottom, has an everted mouth, a lid without handle, a slightly curved spout, four fastenings with four holes on the shoulder, and a flat bottom. On the exterior wall of the teapot the brown pottery body can be seen. The teapot with ordinary workmanship was collected by the museum in 1955 and is basically in good condition.

Preserved in Chinese Medical Association/ Museum of Chinese Medicine, Shanghai University of Traditional Chinese Medicine

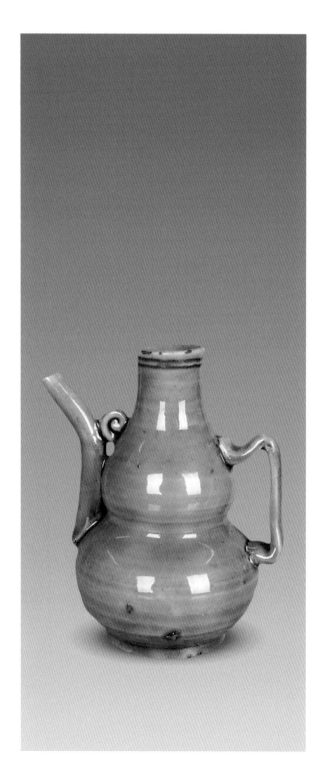

葫芦壶

清

瓷质

口内径 2.25 厘米，口外径 3.95 厘米，底径 7.35 厘米，宽 14.8 厘米，通高 16.8 厘米

Gourd-shaped Kettle

Qing Dynasty

Porcelain

Mouth Inner Diameter 2.25 cm/ Mouth Outer Diameter 3.95 cm/ Bottom Diameter 7.35 cm/ Width 14.8 cm/ Height 16.8 cm

葫芦形。该藏通身施灰绿釉，釉下旋纹明显，圈足平底直口，桥状耳，弯形壶嘴，底无款，工艺粗糙。为饮具。1955 年入藏，保存基本完好。

中华医学会 / 上海中医药大学医史博物馆

The gourd-shaped kettle, which has clear bowstring patterns under the grayish green glaze but no inscription on the bottom, has a vertical mouth, a bridge-shaped handle, a curved spout, and a ring foot. The crude kettle was collected by the museum in 1955 and is basically in good condition.

Preserved in Chinese Medical Association/ Museum of Chinese Medicine, Shanghai University of Traditional Chinese Medicine

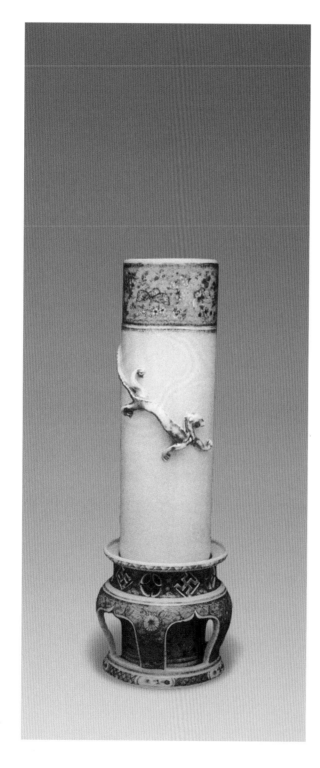

珐琅彩瓷投壶

清

瓷质

通高 48.3 厘米

Enamel Porcelain Pitch-pot

Qing Dynasty

Porcelain

Height 48.3 cm

壶为直筒形，底部置一圆形透雕底座。壶的口沿
和底座部分饰以珐琅彩，壶的中部附一金色的小
龙。此投壶设计华丽，是投壶中的精品。

法国吉美国立亚洲艺术博物馆藏

The cylindrical pitch-pot has a hollowed stand and
a little golden dragon on its middle part. The mouth
rim and the stand are enameled. The pitch-pot looks
gorgeous and is one of the fine pieces of its kind.
Preserved in Musée National des Arts Asiatiques-
Guimet, France

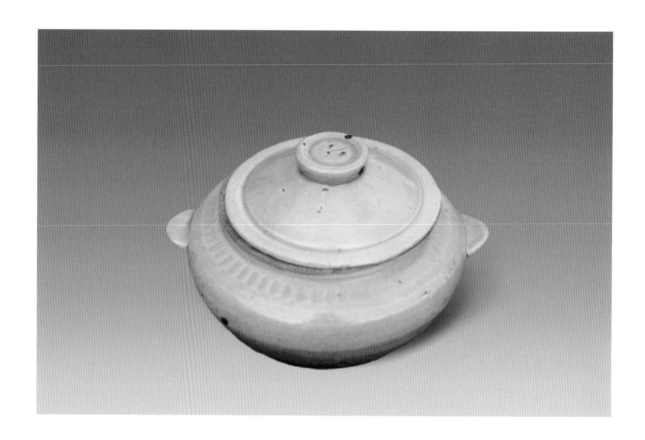

瓷蒸锅带盖

清

瓷质

带盖外口径 15.35 厘米，腹径 20.8 厘米，通高 20 厘米，重 2000 克

Porcelain Steamer Pot with Lid

Qing Dynasty

Porcelain

Mouth Outer Diameter 15.35 cm/ Belly Diameter 20.8 cm/ Total Height 20 cm/ Weight 2,000 g

字母口，溜肩，鼓腹，平底，圈足，带把、带盖蒸锅。用于烹调食物或炖蒸药物。

广东中医药博物馆藏

The porcelain lidded steamer pot has a primary-secondary mouth, a sloping shoulder, a bulged belly, a flat bottom, two handles, and a ring foot. It was used for cooking food or simmering medicinal herbs.

Preserved in Guangdong Chinese Medicine Museum

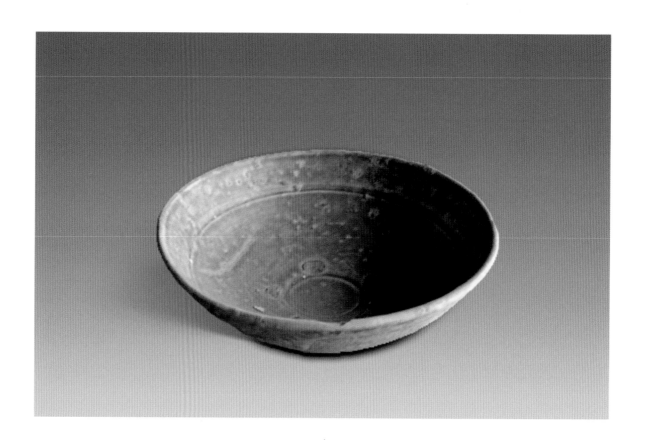

碗

清

瓷质

口径 15 厘米，通高 4.5 厘米

Bowl

Qing Dynasty

Porcelain

Mouth Diameter 15 cm/ Height 4.5 cm

敞口，浅圈足，口稍残，施黄釉。由民间征集。

成都中医药大学中医药传统文化博物馆藏

The yellow-glazed bowl has an everted mouth, a short ring foot, and a slightly damaged mouth. It was collected from a private owner.

Preserved in the Museum of Medicine Preserved in Museum of Traditional Chinese Medicine Culture, Chengdu University of Traditional Chinese Medicine

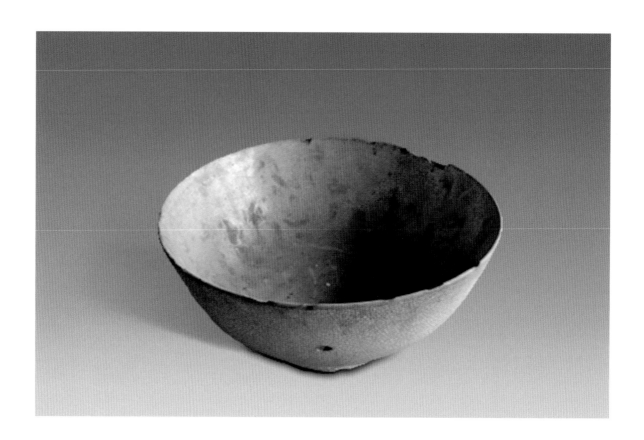

碗

清

瓷质

口径 13.5 厘米，通高 10 厘米

Bowl

Qing Dynasty

Porcelain

Mouth Diameter 13.5 cm/ Height 10 cm

敞口，浅圈足，内施黄釉，外施青釉，有冰
裂纹，口部稍残。由民间征集。

成都中医药大学中医药传统文化博物馆藏

The bowl, painted with yellow glaze on the inside
and cyan glaze on the outside, has an everted
mouth that is slightly damaged, a short ring foot,
and crackled ice patterns on the exterior. It was
collected from a private owner.

Preserved in the Museum of Medicine Preserved
in Museum of Traditional Chinese Medicine
Culture, Chengdu University of Traditional
Chinese Medicine

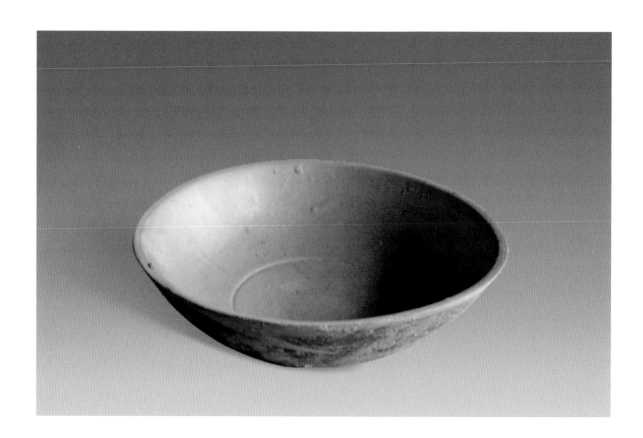

碗

清

瓷质

口径 16 厘米，通高 5 厘米

Bowl

Qing Dynasty

Porcelain

Mouth Diameter 16 cm/ Height 5 cm

敞口，平沿，浅圈足，内施黄釉，外施青釉。
由民间征集。

成都中医药大学中医药传统文化博物馆藏

The bowl, painted with yellow glaze on the
inside and cyan glaze on the outside, has an
everted mouth, a flat rim, and a short ring foot.
It was collected from a private owner.
Preserved in the Museum of Medicine Preserved
in Museum of Traditional Chinese Medicine
Culture, Chengdu University of Traditional
Chinese Medicine

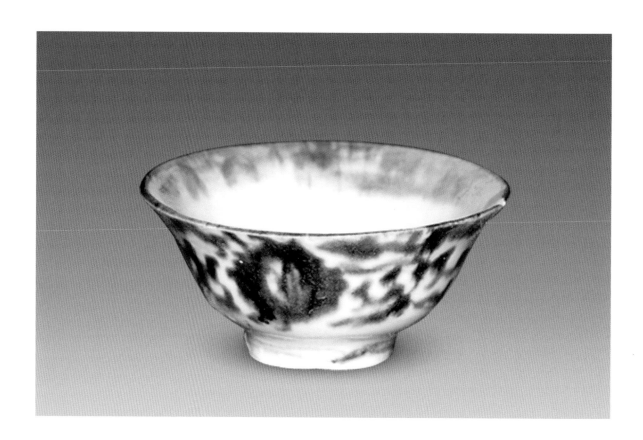

青花小碗

清

瓷质

口径 9.5 厘米，底径 3.6 厘米，通高 4.1 厘米，重 50 克

Small Blue-and-white Bowl

Qing Dynasty

Porcelain

Mouth Diameter 9.5 cm/ Bottom Diameter 3.6 cm/ Height 4.1 cm/ Weight 50 g

敞口，直斜腹，圈足，青花，碗底有一图案，

圈足有一印记。食器，口沿略残。陕西省征集。

陕西医史博物馆藏

The blue-and-white bowl, a tableware, has an
everted mouth that is slightly damaged, a sloping
belly, and a ring foot. There is a pattern on the
bottom and a marking on the ring foot. The bowl
was collected by Shaanxi Province.

Preserved in Shaanxi Museum of Medical History

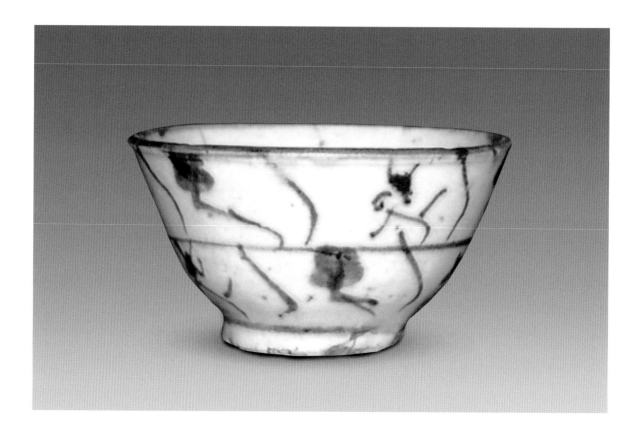

小兰花瓷碗

清

瓷质

口径 10 厘米，底径 4.5 厘米，通高 5 厘米，重 150 克

Porcelain Bowl with Small Orchid Patterns

Qing Dynasty

Porcelain

Mouth Diameter 10 cm/ Bottom Diameter 4.5 cm/ Height 5 cm/ Weight 150 g

敞口，斜腹，圈足，兰花图。食器。碗口有一裂印。

陕西医史博物馆藏

The bowl painted with orchid patterns has an everted mouth, a sloping belly, and a ring foot. There is a crackle near the rim of the tableware.

Preserved in Shaanxi Museum of Medical History

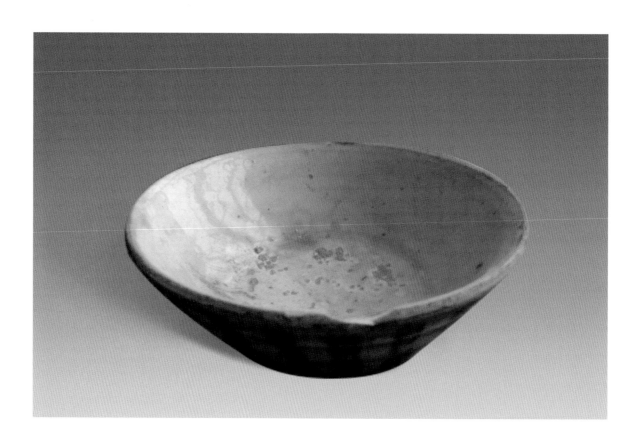

瓷碗

清

瓷质

口径 10.5 厘米，通高 4.2 厘米

Porcelain Bowl

Qing Dynasty

Porcelain

Mouth Diameter 10.5 cm/ Height 4.2 cm

粗瓷小碗。敞口，浅斜腹，圈足，碗内施黄釉，

绘青釉纹，碗外施红釉，有花纹。

江苏省中医药博物馆藏

The bowl, painted with yellow glaze with cyan
lines on the inside and red glaze with decorative
design on the outside, has an everted mouth, a
short tapered belly, and a ring foot. It is made of
crude porcelain.

Preserved in Jiangsu Museum of Traditional
Chinese Medicine

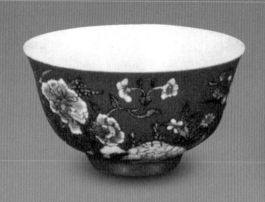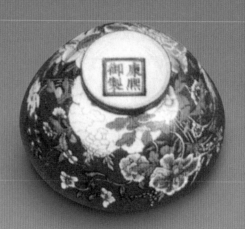

红地珐琅彩瓷碗 一对

清

瓷质

口径 10.8 厘米，底径 4.6 厘米，通高 5 厘米

Pair of Bowls in Enamel Against Vermilion Background

Qing Dynasty

Porcelain

Mouth Diameter 10.8 cm/ Bottom Diameter 4.6 cm/ Height 5 cm

碗内壁和圈足底是纯白釉，底内有堆料青花
年款"康熙御制"四字。碗外壁以朱红色釉
为地，其上用珐琅彩料绘出绿枝蓝花。由于
彩料较厚，图案有立体效果。碗胎坚密而薄，
逆光视之，从碗内可透过光线看到碗外壁的
花纹。清代宫廷御用之器。

广东省博物馆藏

The interior and the ring foot of the bowl are
glazed white. The bottom is inscribed with
four Chinese words "Kang Xi Yu Zhi" (made
in an imperial kiln during Kangxi Reign) in
underglaze blue. There are flowers and branches
in blue and green enamel respectively against
the vermilion background on the exterior wall.
The thick enamel produces a three-dimensional
effect on the patterns. The body is solid but
thin, so from the interior can be seen the flower
patterns on the exterior against light. The
bowl was made in an imperial kiln in the Qing
Dynasty.

Preserved in Guangdong Museum

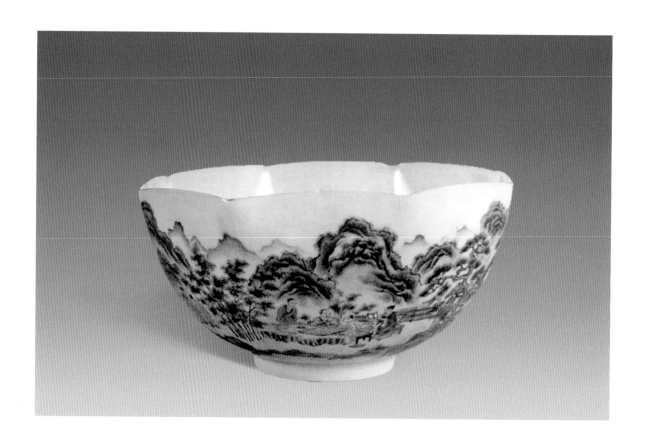

脱抢弈棋粉彩碗

清

瓷质

口径 13.2 厘米，通高 6.9 厘米

Famille Rose Bowl Painted with Men Playing Chinese Chess

Qing Dynasty

Porcelain

Mouth Diameter 13.2 cm/ Height 6.9 cm

碗呈八方委角形，圈足。外壁以山、树为背景，

描绘了两位老者于石桌上摆局对弈的情景。

旁有两人在观棋。

陕西历史博物馆藏

The octagonal bowl with a ring foot is painted
with two old men playing Chinese chess at
a stone table, with two other men behind
watching them and some hills and trees as the
background.

Preserved in Shaanxi History Museum

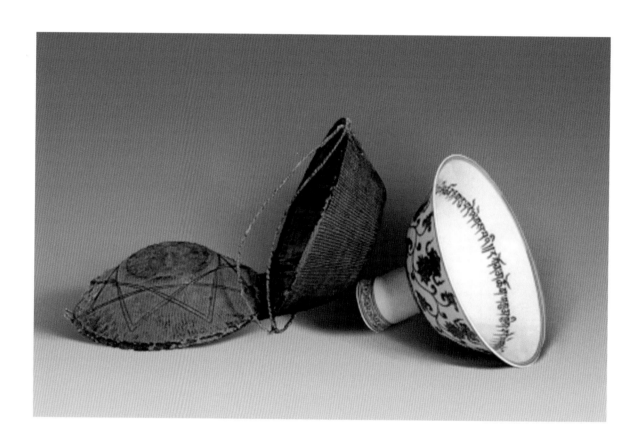

甜白釉缠枝纹高足碗

清

瓷质

口径 14.2 厘米，底部直径 4.2 厘米，足高 4.5 厘米，通高 10 厘米

High-footed Bowl Painted with Intertwining Branches on Sweet White Glaze

Qing Dynasty

Porcelain

Mouth Diameter 14.2 cm/ Bottom Diameter 4.2 cm/ Foot Height 4.5 cm/ Height 10 cm

碗撇口，弧腹，高圈足微外撇。碗内壁绘藏文一周，外壁绘折枝花纹，足绘花纹一周，带碗套。

西藏博物馆藏

The bowl has an everted mouth, an arched belly, and a long slightly flared ring foot. Its interior wall is painted with Tibetan characters in a circle and the exterior wall is painted with intertwining branches. The foot is painted with flower patterns in a circle. There is a cover specially for the bowl.

Preserved in Tibet Museum

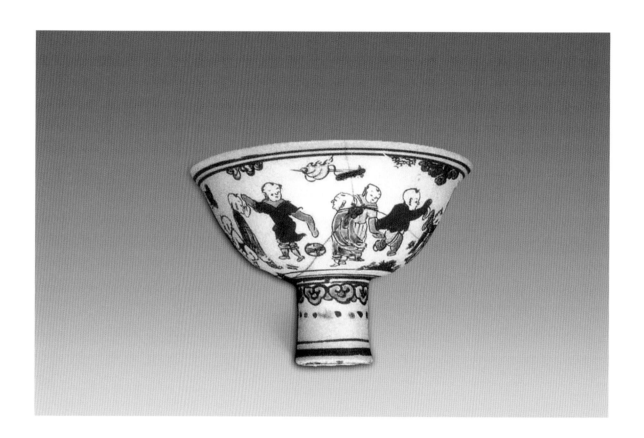

五彩蹴鞠图高足碗

清

瓷质

口径 20 厘米，通高 18.5 厘米

Five-colored High-footed Bowl Painted with Children Playing Cuju Ball

Qing Dynasty

Porcelain

Mouth Diameter 20 cm/ Height 18.5 cm

碗敞口，高足。外壁绘有一组童子进行蹴鞠活动的画面，中间一儿童正甩动双臂欲抬腿踢球，另一位作接球状，旁边有五位伙伴在观看。画面把儿童蹴鞠活动的情形刻画得维妙维肖。

中国体育博物馆藏

The bowl has an everted mouth and a tall foot. The exterior wall is painted with a vivid scene of a group of children playing a cuju ball: one of them flinging his arms is ready to kick the ball, another is about to catch it, and five others are watching them.

Preserved in China Sports Museum

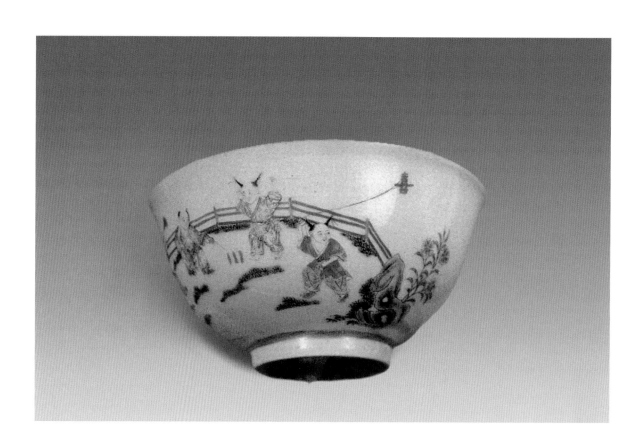

五彩风筝图瓷碗

清

瓷质

口径 25 厘米，通高 15 厘米

Five-colored Porcelain Bowl Painted with Children Flying a Kite

Qing Dynasty

Porcelain

Mouth Diameter 25 cm/ Height 15 cm

碗敞口，圈足。外壁绘有一组童子放风筝的
图案。背景以红、绿等色彩，寥寥数笔绘出
栏杆和树石，给人以轻妙典雅之感。

中国体育博物馆藏

The bowl has an everted mouth and a ring foot.
The exterior wall is painted with a group of
children flying a kite. The background with
balustrade, trees and rocks plainly drawn in red
or green seems relaxing and elegant.

Preserved in China Sports Museum, Beijing

五彩云龙纹碗

清

瓷质

口径 16.7 厘米，底径 7 厘米，通高 8.5 厘米

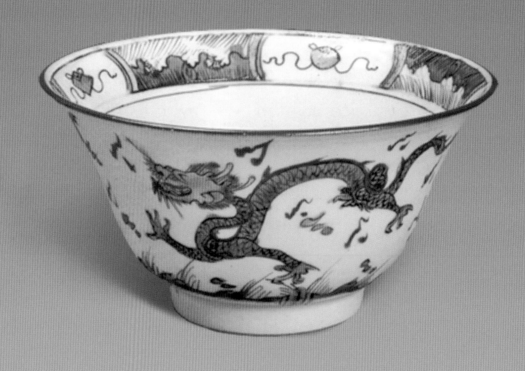

Five-colored Bowl with Dragon and Cloud Patterns

Qing Dynasty

Porcelain

Mouth Diameter 16.7 cm/ Bottom Diameter 7 cm/ Height 8.5 cm

撇口，弧腹，圈足。在白釉上用红、黄、绿、

黑、酱诸彩绘出纹饰。碗心绘火焰纹，口沿

四开光内绘杂宝纹。外壁绘行龙戏珠纹饰。

底白釉署记号款。此碗纹饰生动，色彩缤纷，

当是康熙年间五彩瓷的杰作。

南京市博物馆藏

The bowl has a flared mouth, a sloping belly,

and a ring foot. The bowl is painted with motifs

in red, yellow, green, black and dark reddish

brown on the white glaze: there are flame

motifs on the center of the bowl, motifs of

various treasures enclosed in the four panels

around the mouth rim, dragons chasing a pearl

on the exterior wall, and an inscription against

the white-glazed background on the bottom.

The bowl with vivid and colorful motifs can

be regarded as a masterpiece of five-colored

porcelain ware made during Kangxi Reign of

the Qing Dynasty.

Preserved in Nanjing Museum

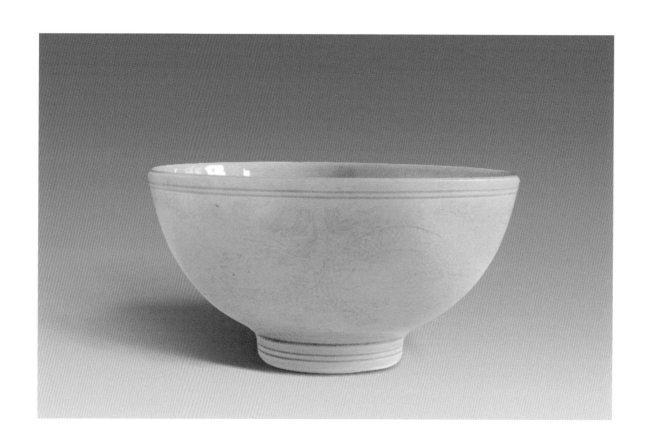

黄釉暗云龙纹碗

清

瓷质

口径 12.5 厘米，通高 8.3 厘米

Yellow-glaze Bowl Incised with Cloud and Dragon Motifs

Qing Dynasty

Porcelain

Mouth Diameter 12.5 cm/ Height 8.3 cm

敞口，鼓腹，圈足。口沿和圈足划暗双弦纹，腹部画暗云龙纹，腹下部饰海水纹，里外施蛋黄色釉，颇匀净，圈足内施白釉，足心青花直书三行"大清道光年制"篆书款，清秀工整，为道光官窑标准款识。

庄锡忠藏

The bowl has an open mouth, a bulged belly, and a ring foot. There are double incised bowstrings near the mouth rim and the ringed foot, incised clouds and a dragon with waves below them on the sides. The bowl is coated with yolk yellow glaze all over, which is even and clean. The interior of the ring foot is glazed with white, against which there are seal-script words "Da Qing Dao Guang Nian Zhi" (made during Daoguang Reign of the Qing Dynasty) in underglaze blue in three lines. The delicate and neat inscription was a standard one of governmental kilns during Daoguang Reign.

Collected by Zhuang Xizhong

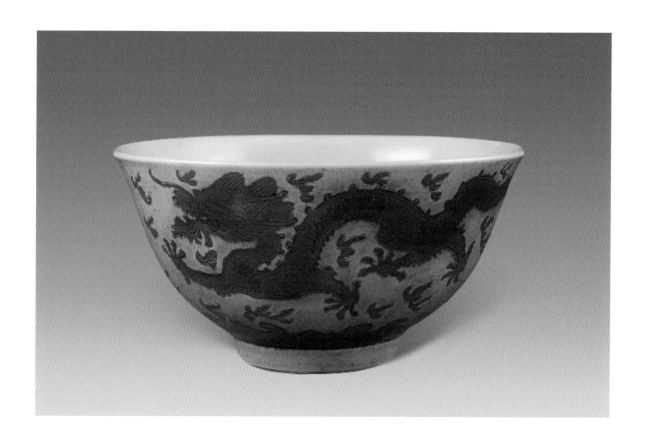

绿地紫彩云龙纹碗

清

瓷质

口径 11.3 厘米，底径 4.3 厘米，通高 5.8 厘米

Bowl Painted with Purple Clouds and Dragon Against Green Background

Qing Dynasty

Porcelain

Mouth Diameter 11.3 cm/ Bottom Diameter 4.3 cm/ Height 5.8 cm

撇口，深腹，圈足。外壁填绿彩为地，绘紫色云龙纹，脚处绘寿山福海纹；底用青花书写"大清道光年制"六字楷书款。应是道光年代官窑作品。

区子谦藏

The bowl has an everted mouth, a deep belly, and a ring foot. There are purple clouds and a dragon against the green background on the exterior, as well as mountains that represent longevity and seas that represent happiness near the foot. Th bottom is inscribed with six regular-script words "Da Qing Dao Guang Nian Zhi" (made during Daoguang Reign of the Qing Dynasty) in underglaze blue. The bowl was probably made in a governmental kiln during Daoguang Reign.

Collected by Qu Ziqian

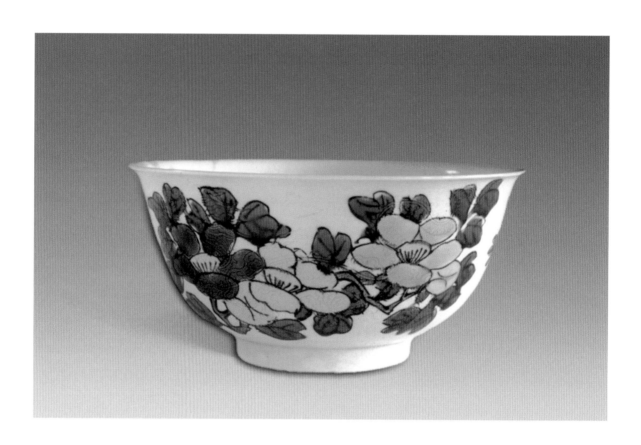

素三彩暗龙纹花蝶碗

清

瓷质

口径 14.9 厘米，底径 6.6 厘米，通高 7 厘米

Three-colored Bowl Incised with Dragon and Painted with Flowers and Butterflies

Qing Dynasty

Porcelain

Mouth Diameter 14.9 cm/ Bottom Diameter 6.6 cm/ Height 7 cm

口微外撇，腹微敛，器形规整，碗身暗绘龙纹，白地，折枝花，瓷质莹润，古朴典雅。

李牧之藏

The regularly-shaped bowl has a slightly everted mouth and a slightly contracted belly. Its body is painted with dark dragon patterns against the white background of plucked flower patterns. The bowl with smooth pottery body is simple but elegant.

Collected by Li Muzhi

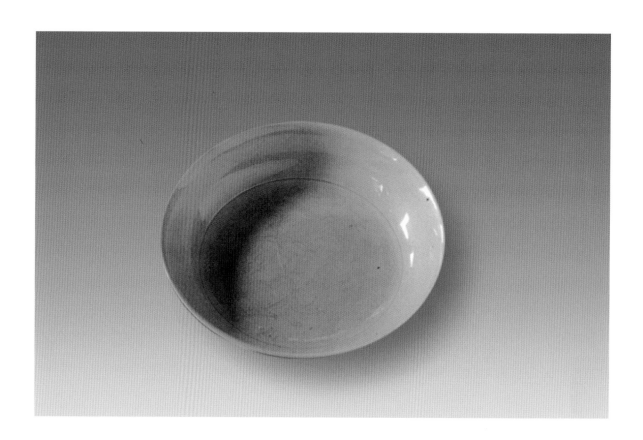

黄釉暗云龙纹盘

清

瓷质

口径 12.8 厘米

Yellow-glazed Dish Incised with Cloud and Dragon Patterns

Qing Dynasty

Porcelain

Mouth Diameter 12.8 cm

敞口，弧形腹，圈足。里外施黄釉，内底刻

云龙纹暗花。圈足内施白釉。足底心画青花

双圈，内直书双行"大清康熙年制"楷书款。

高丰藏

The bowl has an everted mouth, a curved belly,
and a ring foot. It is coated with yellow glaze
all over and incised with clouds and dragons
on the inner center. The white-glazed bottom
is inscribed with six regular-script words "Da
Qing Kang Xi Nian Zhi" (made during Kangxi
Reign of the Qing Dynasty) arranged in two
lines in double circles.

Collected by Gao Feng

粉彩寿山福海纹碗

清

瓷质

口径 12.3 厘米，底径 4.8 厘米，通高 6.5 厘米

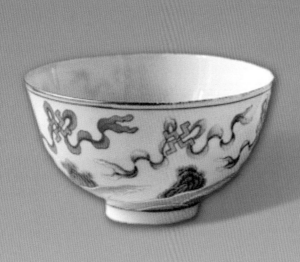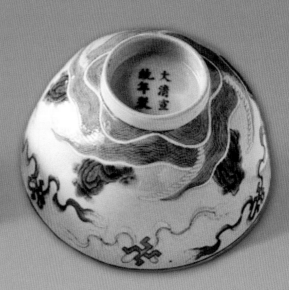

Famille Rose Bowl Pained with Mountains and Seas that Represent Longevity and Good Fortune

Qing Dynasty

Porcelain

Mouth Diameter 12.3 cm/ Bottom Diameter 4.8 cm/ Height 6.5 cm

敞口，深腹，圈足。外壁绘寿山福海捧方胜纹。
底用青花书写"大清宣统年制"六字楷书双
圈款。

谢志峰藏

The bowl has an everted mouth, a deep belly,
and a ring foot. The exterior wall is painted with
mountains that represent longevity and seas that
represent good fortune, and square ornaments.
The bottom is inscribed with regular-script
words "Da Qing Xuan Tong Nian Zhi" (made
during Xuantong Reign of the Qing Dynasty)
enclosed by double rings.

Collected by Xie Zhifeng

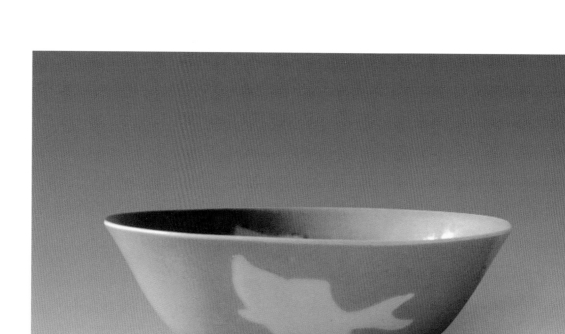

米汤釉白鱼纹碗

清

瓷质

口径 13 厘米

Beige-glazed Bowl with Three Fish Designs

Qing Dynasty

Porcelain

Mouth Diameter 13 cm

撇口，口至足渐收，圈足。外壁腹间饰釉下
白鳜鱼三尾。内壁亦饰白鳜鱼三尾。里外施
米汤釉，温润素雅，与釉里红三鱼碗相比则
别有情趣。底用青花书写"大清康熙年制"
六字楷书款。

高丰藏

The beige-glazed bowl has an everted mouth
that tapers to the ring foot. It is adorned with
three underglazed white fish on the exterior.
The beige glaze is simple but glossy and
elegant, and interesting when compared with
the underglazed red bowl adorned with three
fish. The bottom is inscribed with six regular-
script words "Da Qing Kang Xi Nian Zhi" (made
during Kangxi Reign of the Qing Dynasty) in
underglaze blue.

Collected by Gao Feng

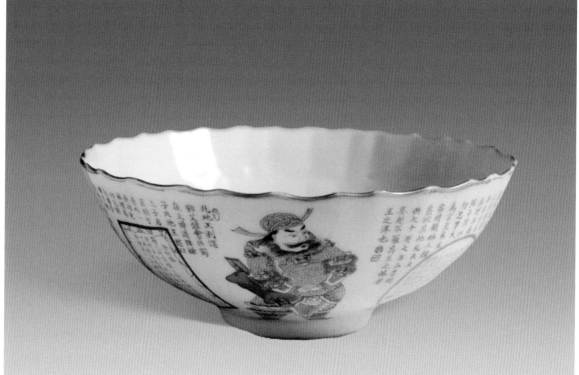

粉彩无双谱瓣口碗

清

瓷质

口径 16.9 厘米，底径 6.1 厘米，通高 6.7 厘米

Multi-lobed Famille Rose Bowl Painted with Album of Unmatched Figures

Qing Dynasty

Porcelain

Mouth Diameter 16.9 cm/ Bottom Diameter 6.1 cm/ Height 6.7 cm

敞口，腹稍鼓，圈足。瓣口施金彩，腹部绘
人物，每一人物以楷书写一小传，相间于四
人物之间，所绘人物精细，楷书工整，似出
于宫廷高手。碗里外施白釉，十分匀净，足
内心书矾红篆书"大清道光年制"六字款。

区子谦藏

The white-glazed bowl has an everted mouth, a
slightly bulged belly, and a ring foot. The multi-
lobed mouth is painted with gold. The belly is
painted with four figures and inscribed with
their brief biographies in regular script; the
figures and biographies are spaced in between.
The figures are delicately painted and the scripts
are neat, so it is possible that they were done by
a master who worked for the imperial family.
The bottom is inscribed with seal-script words
"Da Qing Dao Guang Nian Zhi" (made during
Daoguang Reign of the Qing Dynasty) in iron
red.

Collected by Qu Ziqian

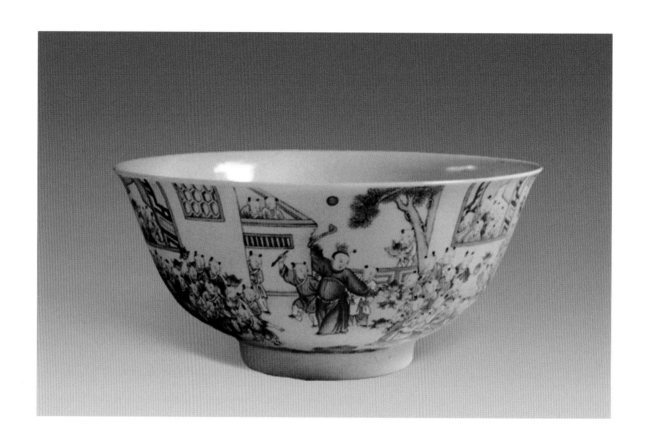

粉彩百子图碗

清

瓷质

口径 18.5 厘米，底径 7.7 厘米，通高 8.4 厘米

Famille Rose Bowl Painted with One Hundred Children

Qing Dynasty

Porcelain

Mouth Diameter 18.5 cm/ Bottom Diameter 7.7 cm/ Height 8.4 cm

撇口，腹稍鼓，圈足。外壁绘儿童百个，故
称百子碗。釉色白而匀净，尚有乾隆余风，
足心书"大清嘉庆年制"六字篆书方款。

区子谦藏

The bowl has an everted mouth, a slightly
bulged belly, and a ring foot. It is painted with
one hundred children on the exterior. As one
hundred children is called "Baizi" in Chinese,
the bowl is called "Baizi bowl". The white
glaze is even and clean and still more or less
keeps the characteristics of those made during
Qianlong Reign. The bottom is inscribed
with Chinese words "Da Qing Jia Qing Nian
Zhi" (made during Jiaqing Reign of the Qing
Dynasty) in seal script.

Collected by Qu Ziqian

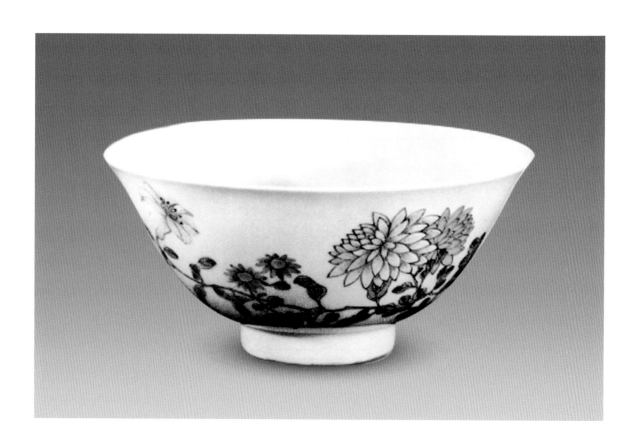

粉彩折枝花卉纹碗

清

瓷质

口径 14.5 厘米，通高 6.1 厘米

Famille Rose Bowl Painted with Plucked Flower Patterns

Qing Dynasty

Porcelain

Mouth Diameter 14.5 cm/ Height 6.1 cm

此碗胎体处理非常讲究，光滑细腻，洁白无
瑕，图案也极为传神，这是雍正粉彩瓷的特
点。底足有"大清雍正年制"的题款。常用
作餐具。

首都博物馆藏

The bowl was a common tableware. The pottery
body was delicately processed: it is fine, smooth
and snowy, and the patterns are lifelike, both
characterizing the famille rose porcelain ware
made during Yongzheng Reign. The bottom is
inscribed with Chinese words "Da Qing Yong
Zheng Nian Zhi" (made during Yongzheng
Reign of the Qing Dynasty).

Preserved in the Capital Museum

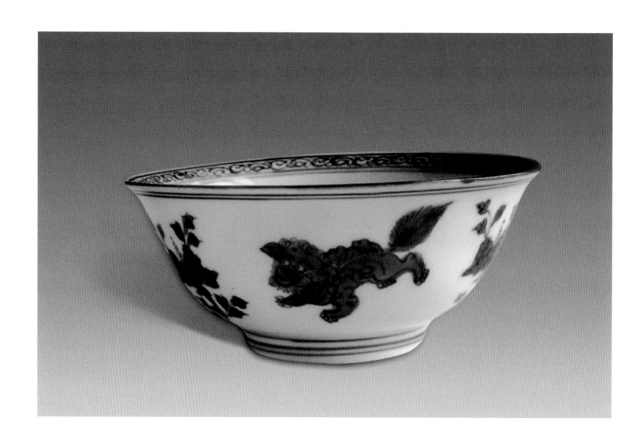

青花狮子花卉纹碗

清

瓷质

口径 14.5 厘米，底径 6.2 厘米，通高 5.9 厘米

Blue-and-white Bowl Painted with Lions and Flower Motifs

Qing Dynasty

Porcelain

Mouth Diameter 14.5 cm/ Bottom Diameter 6.2 cm/ Height 5.9 cm

敞口，深腹，圈足。碗内口缘绘一周卷草纹，中央绘折枝花；外壁绘三只狮子纹，间以折枝花。底书写"大明嘉靖年制"六字楷书款。青花色浓艳，白釉闪青，应是雍正年制品。

李志峰藏

The bowl has an everted mouth, a deep belly, and a ring foot. There is a circle of scroll patterns around the inner rim, plucked flower patterns on the center, and three lions and plucked flower motifs spaced in between on the exterior wall. The bottom is inscribed with six regular-script words "Da Qing Jia Jing Nian Zhi" (made during Jiajing Rein of the Ming Dynasty). The bowl is supposed to have been made during Yongzheng Reign of the Qing Dynasty as the patterns are bright-colored and the white glaze takes on a shade of cyan.

Collected by Li Zhifeng

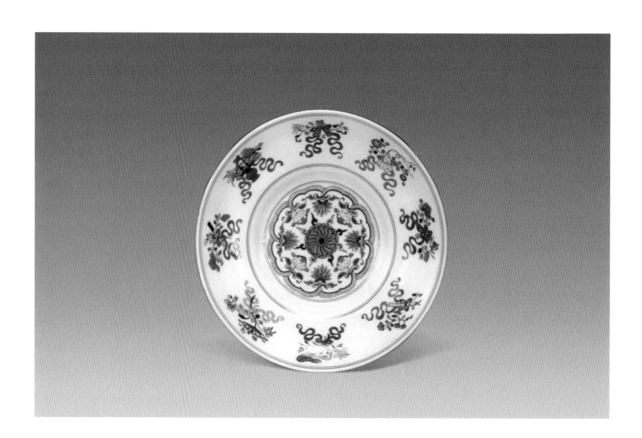

斗彩缠枝花卉暗八仙纹碗

清

瓷质

口径 22 厘米，底径 10.1 厘米，通高 5.3 厘米

Doucai Bowl Painted with Intertwining Flower Motifs and Talismans of the Eight Immortals

Qing Dynasty

Porcelain

Mouth Diameter 22 cm/ Bottom Diameter 10.1 cm/ Height 5.3 cm

侈口，腹壁上弧下直，折腰，大圈足，白釉厚底。周身均用斗彩装饰，外壁为缠枝花卉和如意云纹间仰莲纹；碗心饰一轮花，内壁绘暗八仙纹，即道教中八仙手持之物花篮、阴阳板、葫芦、宝剑、道情筒、扇子、荷花、笛子。足底青花六字三行篆款"大清乾隆年制"。

常州市博物馆藏

The mouth of the bowl is flared and the foot is big and round. The upper part of the belly is curved, the middle part is straight, and the lower part is sloping. Against the heavy white glaze on the bowl there are doucai patterns: intertwining flower, ruyi cloud motifs and upright lotus patterns on the exterior wall; a wheel-like floral motif on the center; and talismans of the Eight Immortals, namely, flower basket, yin & yang panel, gourd, treasure sword, musical instrument used by Daoists for preaching, fan, lotus and flute, on the interior wall. The bottom of the bowl is inscribed with underglaze blue with six seal-script words "Da Qing Qian Long Nian Zhi" (made during Qianlong Reign of the Qing Dynasty) arranged in three rows.

Preserved in Changzhou Museum

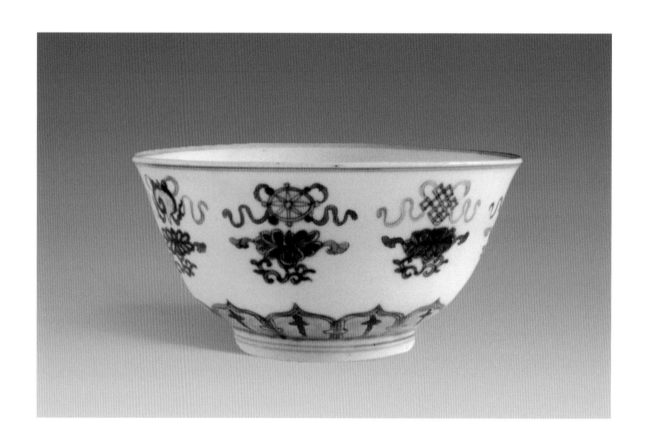

斗彩八宝纹碗

清

瓷质

口径 17 厘米，底径 8.2 厘米，通高 8.5 厘米

Doucai Bowl Painted with Eight Treasures

Qing Dynasty

Porcelain

Mouth Diameter 17 cm/ Bottom Diameter 8.2 cm/ Height 8.5 cm

敞口稍外撇，由口至下渐收，圈足。口沿和足上部各画双弦纹一道，外壁绘八宝一周，腹下画变形莲瓣纹，内沿和近底处各画双弦纹一道。施白釉稍泛青色，白净明亮，纹饰简约疏朗，为清早期绘瓷的特点。

蓝子杏藏

The bowl has a slightly everted mouth, a contracted belly, and a ring foot. There are double bowstrings around the rim on the exterior and interior, above the foot, and near the center of the bowl. Eight treasures are painted on the exterior wall and distorted lotus petal motifs on the lower part of the belly. The bluish white glaze is clean and bright, and the patterns are concise and relaxing, characterizing the porcelain patterns of the Early Qing Dynasty.

Collected by Lan Zixing

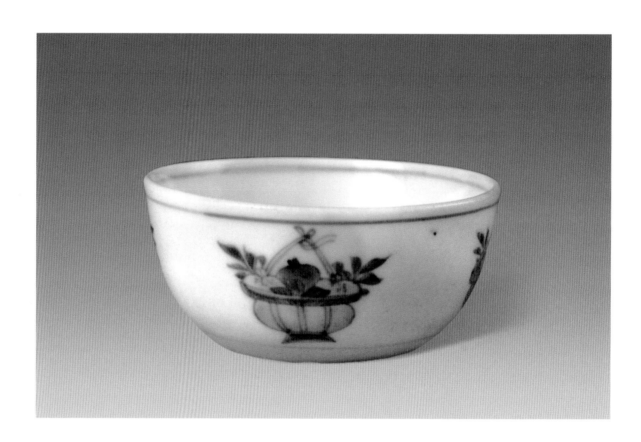

斗彩花篮纹墩式碗

清

瓷质

口径 6 厘米

Drum-shaped Doucai Bowl Painted with Flower Baskets

Qing Dynasty

Porcelain

Mouth Diameter 6 cm

直口，腹微敛，凹底无釉，胎质细腻。外壁
纹饰分两层，腹部绘一组花篮纹，内底绘变
形花篮纹，纹饰精细生动，制作考究。

杜灿佳藏

The exquisite bowl has a vertical mouth, a
slightly contracted belly, and an unglazed
concave base. The fine exterior wall is
decorated with a group of flower baskets and
the interior bottom is painted with a group of
distorted flower baskets, which are delicate and
vivid.

Collected by Du Canjia

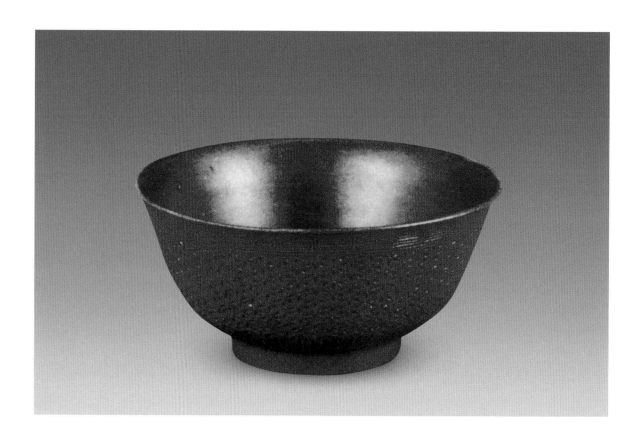

仿雕漆碗

清

瓷质

口径 12.5 厘米，底径 5.7 厘米

Porcelain Bowl Imitated from Carved Lacquered Ware

Qing Dynasty

Porcelain

Mouth Diameter 12.5 cm/ Bottom Diameter 5.7 cm

大口深腹，高圈足，造型古朴端庄。碗内壁在胎体上均匀涂抹一层金光闪闪的釉，颇似古铜，又像鎏金。外壁雕出云雷纹、花瓣纹和莲花纹，以朱红为基本色调，与内壁的深黄极为协调，反映了这一时期仿制工艺水平的高超。

广东省博物馆藏

The bowl has a wide mouth, a deep belly, and a tall ring foot. It looks simple and solemn. The interior wall is evenly covered with glittering golden glaze, which particularly looks like archaic bronze or gilding. The exterior wall is carved with cloud and thunder patterns, petal and lotus motifs, of which vermilion is the basic tone, which harmonizes with the dark yellow on the interior wall. These reflect that the imitation technique had reached a high level in that period.

Preserved in Guangdong Museum

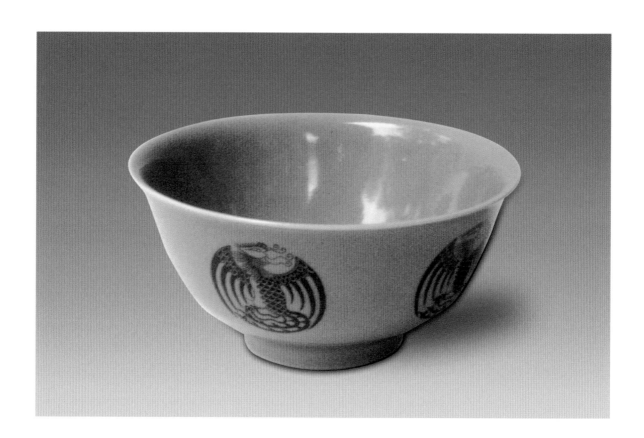

冬青釉抹红团凤纹碗

清

瓷质

口径 14 厘米，通高 7 厘米

Bowl Painted with Red Rounded Phoenixes on Holly Green Glaze

Qing Dynasty

Porcelain

Mouth Diameter 14 cm/ Height 7 cm

撇口渐往下收，腹鼓，圈足。外满施匀净的
冬青釉，里和底施白釉，腹间以抹红绘团凤
四只，呈色鲜艳稳定。圈足内心有篆书"大
清乾隆年制"六字款。此种碗乾隆、道光时
多见，碗形典雅美观。

李明藏

The bowl has an everted mouth and a bulged belly that tapers to the ring foot. There are four red rounded phoenixes against the holly green glaze on the exterior wall; the red color is bright and even. The white-glazed bottom is inscribed with six seal-script words "Da Qing Qian Long Nian Zhi" (made during Qianlong Reign of the Qing Dynasty). This type of elegant and beautiful bowl was very common during Qianlong and Daoguang Reigns.

Collected by Li Ming

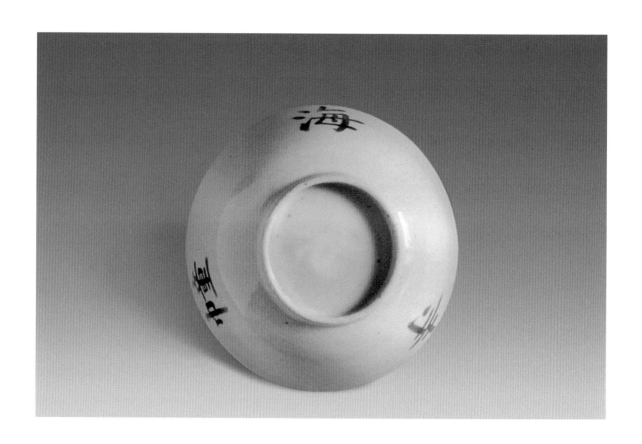

白釉矾红 "海幢寺" 款碗

清

瓷质

口径 14 厘米，足径 6.5 厘米，通高 6.5 厘米

White-glazed Bowl Inscribed with "Hoi Tong Monastery" in Iron Red

Qing Dynasty

Porcelain

Mouth Diameter 14 cm/ Foot Diameter 6.5 cm/ Height 6.5 cm

敞口，深腹，圈足。外壁用矾红色书写"海幢寺"

楷书品字形三字，这是广州和河南"海幢寺"

和尚当时所用之物。该碗也称"澹归碗"，

是因当时澹归和尚自资烧造之物而得名。

赵汉光藏

The bowl has an everted mouth, a deep belly, and a ring foot. The exterior wall is inscribed with three regular-script words "Honam Temple" in " 品 " (pin) shape. This kind of bowl was used by Buddhist monks of Hoi Tong Monastery in Guangzhou City and Henan Province. The bowl is also called "Dangui Bowl", for it was Buddhist monk Dangui who paid for the bowls to be made.

Collected by Zhao Hanguang

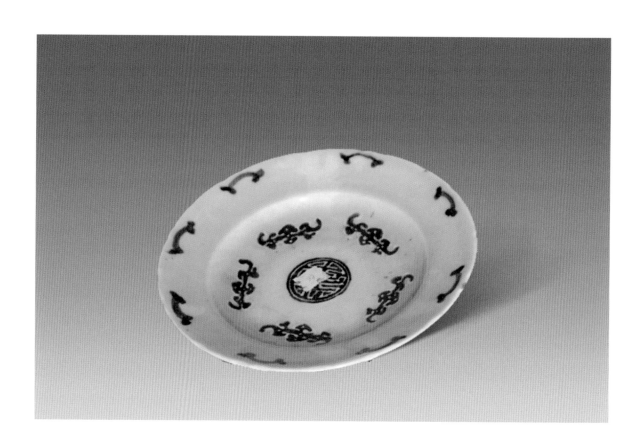

豆绿大瓷盘

清

瓷质

口径 26 厘米，底径 12.5 厘米，通高 5 厘米，重 800 克

Porcelain Plate Glazed Bean Green

Qing Dynasty

Porcelain

Mouth Diameter 26 cm/ Bottom Diameter 12.5 cm/ Height 5 cm/ Weight 800 g

盘足，圈足，豆绿色小兰花，图案盘中有一"寿"字，盘底有"成化年制"。食器。完整无损。

陕西医史博物馆藏

The plate has a ring foot, tiny bean green orchid motifs on the exterior, the word "Shou" (longevity) on the center, and "Cheng Hua Nian Zhi" (made during Chenghua Period) on the bottom. The tableware is in good condition.

Preserved in Shaanxi Museum of Medical History

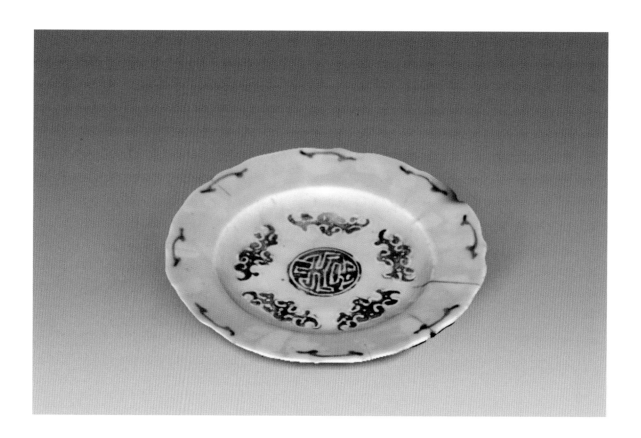

绿釉瓷盘

清

瓷质

口径 26 厘米，底径 12.5 厘米，通高 4 厘米，重 900g

Green-glazed Plate

Qing Dynasty

Porcelain

Mouth Diameter 26 cm/ Bottom Diameter 12.5 cm/ Height 4 cm/ Weight 900 g

口呈花边形，盘内五蝠棒"寿"图，圈足。食器。
盘口有裂印。

陕西医史博物馆藏

The plate has a petal-shaped rim, a ring foot, and
five bats around the word "Shou" (longevity) on
the center. There are cracles on the mouth rim of
the tableware.

Preserved in Shaanxi Museum of Medical History

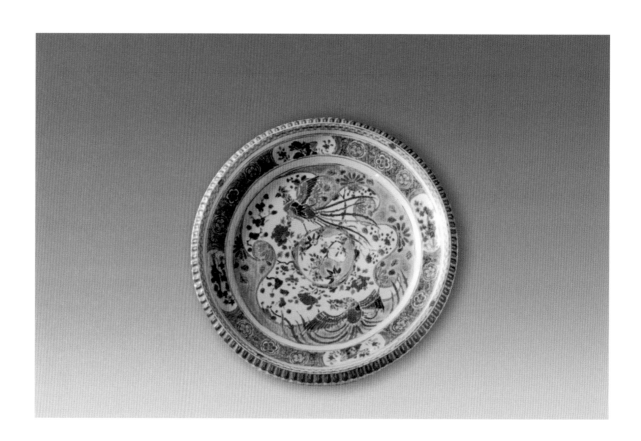

五彩凤纹大盘

清

瓷质

口径 52 厘米

Famille Verte Plate Painted with Phoenix Designs

Qing Dynasty

Porcelain

Mouth Diameter 52 cm

折缘，浅腹，圈足。花口绘菊花瓣纹，内壁绘开窗鱼，虾对称纹，间以梅花纹，盘中央绘双凤穿牡丹花。彩色鲜艳，白釉莹润，是康熙时期民窑佳作。

高丰藏

The shallow plate with chrysanthemum petal-shaped rim and a ring foot is painted with fish and shrimps enclosed in four panels spaced by four groups of plum blossoms on the interior wall, and a pair of phoenixes among peonies on the center. The plate with colorful painting and glossy white glaze is an excellent piece made in a non-official kiln during Kangxi Reign of the Qing Dynasty.

Collected by Gao Feng

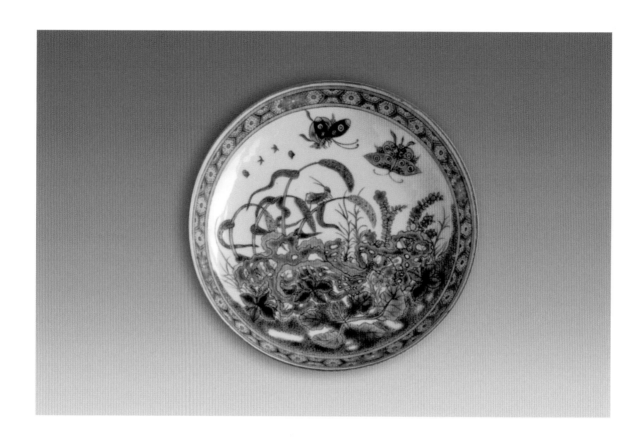

五彩花蝶纹盘

清

瓷质

口径 14 厘米，底径 8.5 厘米，通高 2.5 厘米

Famille Verte Plate Painted with Flower and Butterfly Motifs

Qing Dynasty

Porcelain

Mouth Diameter 14 cm/ Bottom Diameter 8.5 cm/ Height 2.5 cm

敞口，浅腹，圈足。盘内口缘绿地，绘朵花纹；

盘内中央绘花卉飞蝶等纹饰。金底红彩书写

"玉清书屋"四字楷书款。

舒浩光藏

The plate has an everted mouth, a shallow belly, and a ring foot. The inner mouth rim is decorated with flower patterns on the green glaze. The inner center is painted with butterflies fluttering among flowers. The bottom is inscribed with four regular-script red words "Yu Qing Shu Wu" indicating a study named Yu Qing against the golden background.

Collected by Shu Haoguang

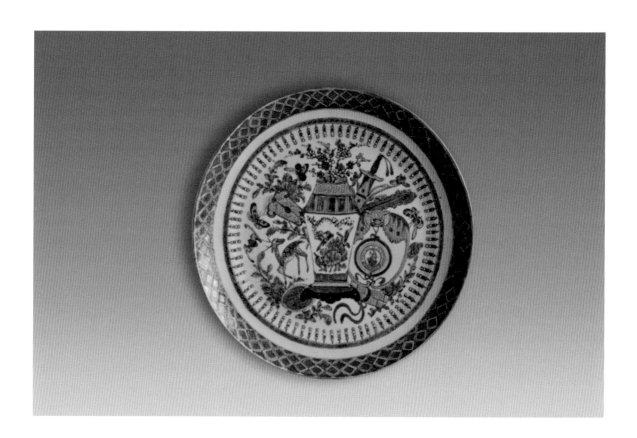

广彩花卉盘

清

瓷质

口径 26 厘米，底径 16.5 厘米

Guangzhou-overglazed Plate Painted with Flower Motifs

Qing Dynasty

Porcelain

Mouth Diameter 26 cm/ Bottom Diameter 16.5 cm

撇口，浅腹，圈足。盘中央绘一花瓶，内插折枝梅花，瓶周围绘花蝶、蝙蝠、鹿纹与两件八宝纹饰，其外绘璎珞纹一周，口缘红地绘斜方格纹，底用矾红书写"宣统年宝兴造"及英文。

张家光藏

The shallow dish has an everted mouth and a ring foot. On its center is a vase with several plucked plum blossoms in it, which is surrounded by motifs of butterflies, bats, deer and two treasures, which are enclosed by a circle of tassels. There is a reticulate scroll against the red background around the rim. The bottom is inscribed with six Chinese characters "Xuan Tong Nian Bao Xing Zao" (made in Baoxing during Xuantong Reign) and their English version in iron red.

Collected by Zhang Jiaguang

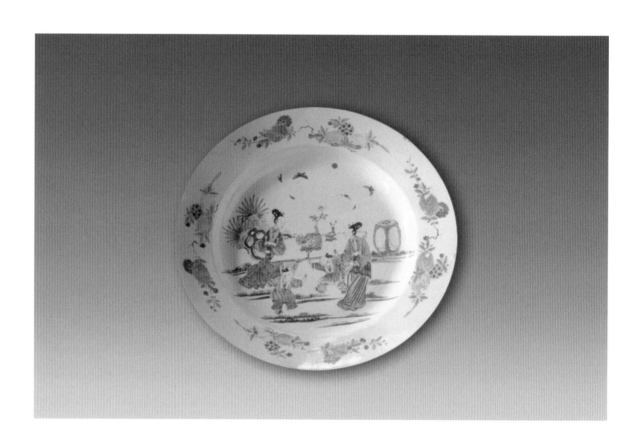

粉彩母婴纹板沿盘

清

瓷质

口径 20.3 厘米

Famille Rose Plate with Flattened Rim and Patterns of Mothers and Children

Qing Dynasty

Porcelain

Mouth Diameter 20.3 cm

板沿，折腰，浅圈足，圈足内直外斜。底施白釉较薄，可见旋轮痕迹。板沿绘石榴、佛手等吉祥如意花果。盘内画母子婴戏图，两仕女各带一婴儿在庭园内玩耍，形神兼备，构图新颖，彩色艳丽，应为康熙晚期民窑的佳作。

高丰藏

The plate has a flattened rim, a sloped belly, and a short ring foot that is straight inside and sloping outside. The bottom is covered with relatively thin white glaze, from which can be seen scratches of the spinning roller. On the flattened rim there are pomegranates, bergamots and some other fruits that represent good fortune and happiness. The center of the plate is painted with two ladies playing with each of their children in the garden. There is a perfect unity between their appearances and facial expressions. The composition is novel and the colors are bright. The plate can be rated as an excellent one among those made in non-governmental kilns during Kangxi Reign of the Qing Dynasty.

Collected by Gao Feng

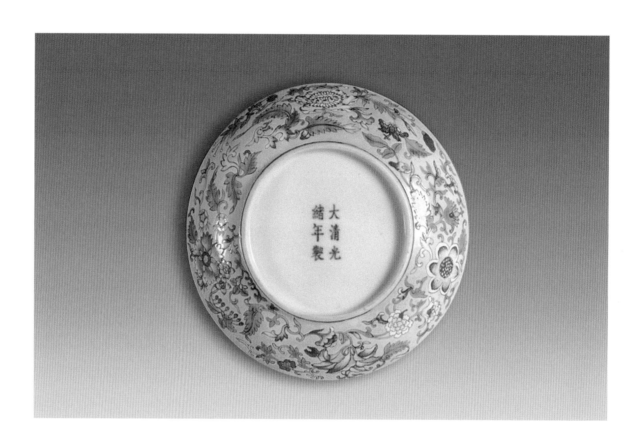

粉彩花卉盘

清

瓷质

口径 20.5 厘米

Famille Rose Plate Painted with Flower Motifs

Qing Dynasty

Porcelain

Mouth Diameter 20.5 cm

敞口，浅腹，圈足。外壁以黄色为地，绘折枝花，彩色鲜艳。底用青花书写"大清光绪年制"六字楷书款。这是光绪官窑代表作。

梁权藏

The shallow dish has an open mouth and a ring foot. There are bright plucked flower patterns against the yellow background on the exterior wall. The bottom is inscribed with six regular-script words "Da Qing Guang Xu Nian Zhi" (made during Guangxu Reign of the Qing Dynasty) in underglaze blue. The plate is a representative one among those made in governmental kilns during Guangxu Reign of the Qing Dynasty.

Collected by Liang Quan

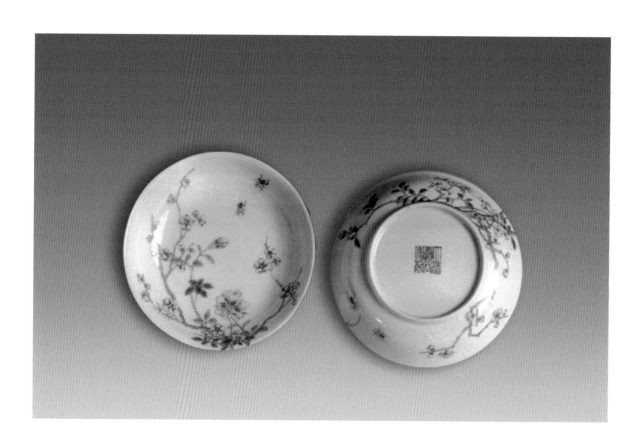

粉彩过墙花卉纹盘

清

瓷质

口径 11.8 厘米

Famille Rose Plate Painted with Successive Flower Motifs

Qing Dynasty

Porcelain

Mouth Diameter 11.8 cm

敞口，弧形腹，圈足。里外施白釉，外壁和内里均画花卉，两两相联，名曰过墙花，粉彩淡雅清秀，道光朝多此画法。底心红彩篆书"大清道光年制"六字方款。该盘是道光官窑的代表作。

梁奕嵩藏

The plate has an open mouth, a curved belly, and a ring foot. The floral motifs are called "Guo Qiang Hua" in Chinese meaning flowers that climb over the wall, for the motifs on the interior wall are connected with those on the exterior, a technique that was common during Daoguang Reign. The famille rose palette is elegant, delicate and pretty. The center of the bottom is inscribed with six red seal-script words "Da qing Dao Guang Nian Zhi" (made during Daoguang Reign of the Qing Dynasty). The plate was a representative one among those made in governmental kilns of Daoguang Reign.

Collected by Liang Yisong

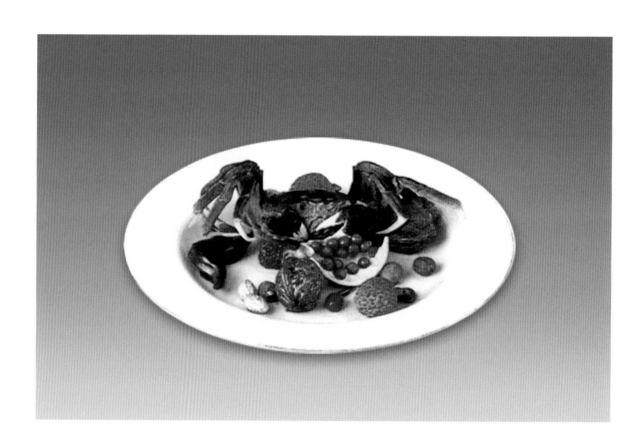

粉彩果品盘

清

瓷质

口径 22 厘米，足径 12.3 厘米，通高 6.5 厘米

Famille Rose Fruit Plate

Qing Dynasty

Porcelain

Mouth Diameter 22 cm/ Foot Diameter 12.3 cm/ Height 6.5 cm

盘沿宽而外折，腹深而直，圈足。通体施白釉，口部描金。盘内粘接有瓷塑的一只肥蟹，周围是荔枝、樱桃、红枣、核桃、花生、瓜子、石榴等瓜果类食品。盘中瓷塑食品均采用平涂施彩的方法，根据食品种类、形态的不同分别施彩，极其形象逼真，代表了乾隆时期像生瓷制作的高超技艺。

故宫博物院藏

The plate has a flattened rim, a deep belly, and a ring foot. It is coated with white glaze all over and the rim is smeared with gold. The plate is connected with a big porcelain scrab, which is surrounded by porcelain litchis, cherries, jujubes, walnuts, peanuts, watermelon seeds and pomegranate. The fruits are smeared with different colors according to their sorts and shapes. The vivid fruits embody the superb manufacturing technique of true-to-life porcelain ware during Qianlong Reign of the Qing Dynasty.

Preserved in the Palace Museum

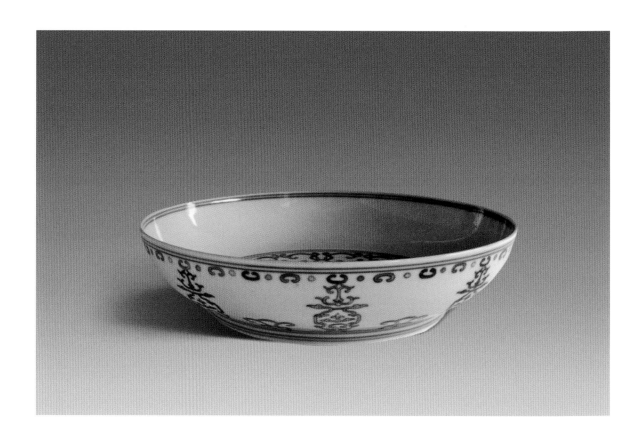

斗彩寿字纹盘

清

瓷质

口径 21 厘米，底径 13.5 厘米，通高 4.9 厘米

Doucai Plate Adorned with Longevity-representing Patterns

Qing Dynasty

Porcelain

Mouth Diameter 21 cm/ Bottom Diameter 13.5 cm/ Height 4.9 cm

敞口，深腹，圈足。盘中彩绘如意头纹，中央为一寿字纹，周围八寿字纹；外壁也绘八寿字纹。底用青花书写"大清道光年制"六字篆书款。胎坚细，釉莹白，器底白釉现波浪纹，略闪青。这是道光官窑代表作。

章兆泉藏

The plate has an open mouth, a deep belly, and a ring foot. There are Ruyi heads on the plate, a " 寿 " (Shou) pattern (Shou in pinyin, a word meaning longevity) surrounded by eight " 寿 " (Shou) patterns on the center, eight "寿" (Shou) patterns on the exterior wall, and underglaze blue inscriptions "Da Qing Dao Guang Nian Zhi" (made during Daoguang Reign of the Qing Dynasty) in seal script on the bottom. The pottery body is hard, solid and fine; the white glaze is glossy; and the white glaze on the bottom is slightly bluish with wave patterns. The plate was a representative one made in a governmental kiln during Daoguang Reign.

Collected by Zhang Zhaoquan

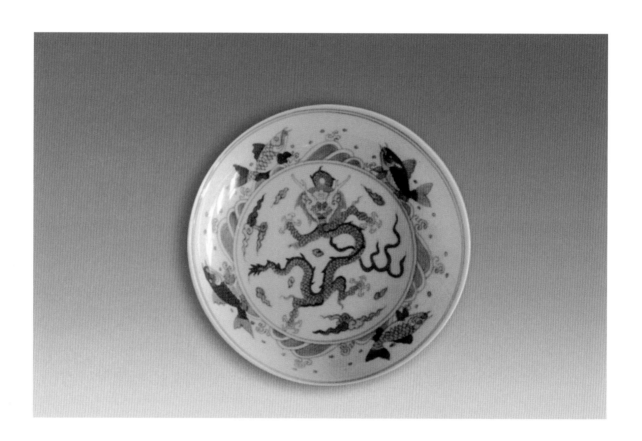

斗彩云龙鱼纹盘

清

瓷质

口径 15.3 厘米，底径 9.1 厘米，通高 3.5 厘米

Doucai Plate Painted with Cloud, Dragon and Fish Motifs

Qing Dynasty

Porcelain

Mouth Diameter 15.3 cm/ Bottom Diameter 9.1 cm/ Height 3.5 cm

敞口、稍内收，弧形腹，圈足。沿内和内壁下各画双弦纹一道，内壁绘海水游鱼四条，内底画正面龙云纹，整个画面配合得当，生动有致。里外施白釉，白中稍泛青，晶莹明亮。足内楷书"成化年制"款，尚有雍正笔意，实为雍正仿成化斗彩之作。

高成藏

The plate has a slightly contracted open mouth, a curved belly, and a ring foot. There are double rounded bowstrings near the rim and below the interior wall, four fish roving about the sea on the interior wall, and a dragon among clouds on the inner center. The whole picture is lively and properly arranged. The white glaze that covers the interior and exterior is bluish, bright and glossy. The regular-script words on the base "Cheng Hua Nian Zhi" (made during Chenghua Period) follow Emperor Yongzheng's calligraphic style, indicating that the dish was an imitation of a Doucai porcelain made during Chenghua Period of the Ming Dynasty.
Collected by Gao Cheng

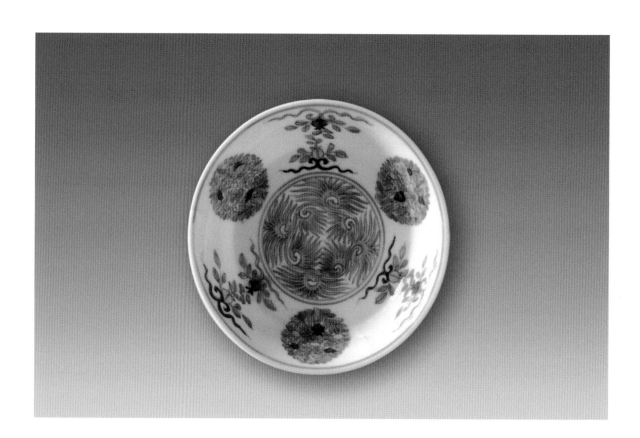

斗彩花卉盘

清

瓷质

口径 21 厘米

Doucai Plate Painted with Flower Motifs

Qing Dynasty

Porcelain

Mouth Diameter 21 cm

撇口，沿稍折，圈足。外壁口沿划双弦纹，近足处亦划弦纹一道，内绘三折枝花，匀称地饰于盘外壁上。内壁绘团花和折枝花相间，口沿画弦纹一道，底心于双道弦纹内画水草纹。底足青花双圈。

高丰藏

The plate has an everted mouth and a ring foot. On the exterior wall there are double bowstrings around the rim, a bowstring near the foot, double rings in underglaze blue on the base, and three plucked flower motifs spaced evenly on the wall. The interior wall is decorated with a bowstring around the rim, plucked flower branches and clustered flowers spaced in between, and water plants enclosed by double rings on the center.

Collected by Gao Feng

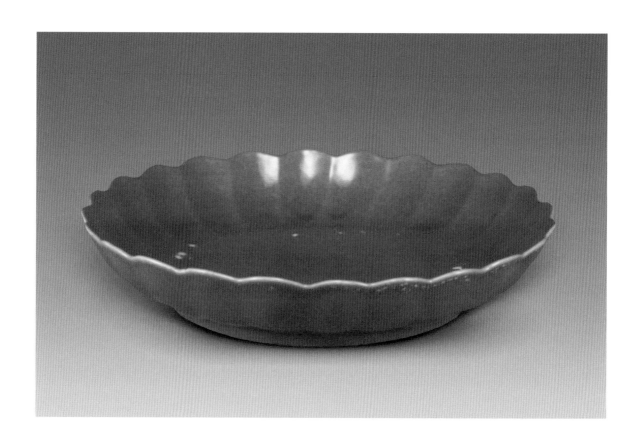

胭脂红釉菊瓣形盘

清

瓷质

口径 16.2 厘米，底径 10.5 厘米，通高 3 厘米

Chrysanthemum Petal-shaped Plate in Carmine Glaze

Qing Dynasty

Porcelain

Mouth Diameter 16.2 cm/ Bottom Diameter 10.5 cm/ Height 3 cm

盘为二十四出菊瓣形,内外壁均施胭脂红釉,

发色鲜艳,宽圈足,足墙内收,盘心微凹。

白釉底书六字双行青花楷书款"大清雍正年

制",外围双圈。

常州市博物馆藏

The slightly hollow plate has 24 chrysanthemum petal-shaped sides and a big and contracted ring foot. It is coated with bright carmine glaze all over. The white-glazed bottom is inscribed with six regular-script words "Da Qing Yong Zheng Nian Zhi" (made during Yongzheng Reign of the Qing Dynasty) in underglaze blue, in two lines surrounded by double rings.

Preserved in Changzhou Museum

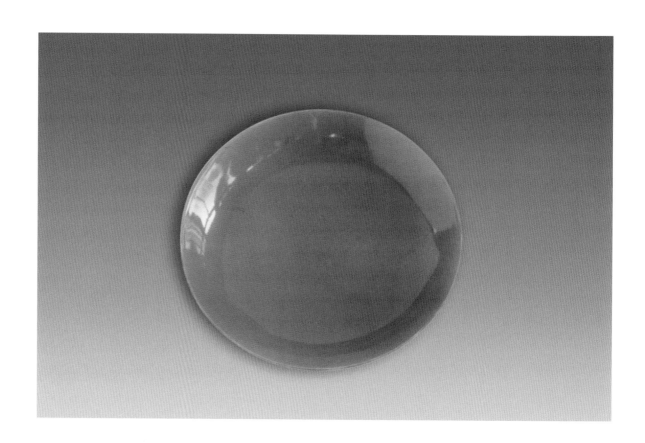

胭脂红盘

清

瓷质

口径 16.7 厘米，通高 3.3 厘米

Carmine-glazed Plate

Qing Dynasty

Porcelain

Mouth Diameter 16.7 cm/ Height 3.3 cm

敞口，弧形腹，圈足。外壁施浅绿色釉，内里施胭脂红釉，虽无甚纹饰，红绿相映，却显得特别娇嫩美观。足内施白釉，中心两行青花楷书"大清光绪年制"款。

李庆全藏

The plate has an open mouth, a curved belly, and a ring foot. The exterior wall is coated with light green glaze while the interior wall is coated with carmine glaze. Although there is no pattern, the green and the carmine colors harmonize with each other, making the plate pretty and delicate. The interior of the ring foot is glazed white and inscribed with regular-script words "Da Qing Guang Xu Nian Zhi" (made during Guangxu Reign of the Qing Dynasty) in underglaze blue in two lines.

Collected by Li Qingquan

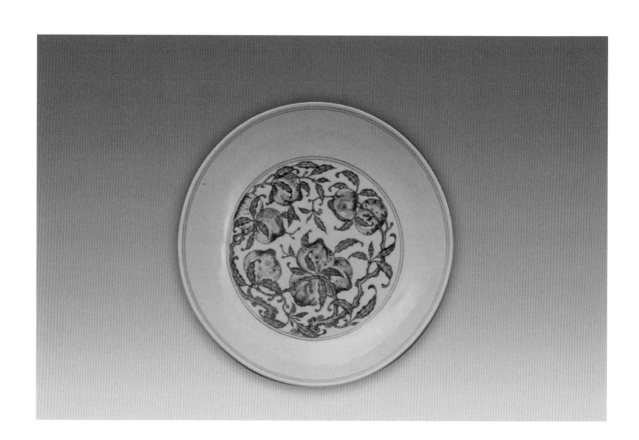

黄釉青花缠枝九桃盘

清

瓷质

口径 27 厘米，底径 17.5 厘米，通高 5.1 厘米

Yellow-glazed Plate Painted with Nine Blue-and-white Peaches and Intertwining Branches

Qing Dynasty

Porcelain

Mouth Diameter 27 cm/ Bottom Diameter 17.5 cm/ Height 5.1 cm

敞口，浅弧腹，圈足。盘心有青花绘九桃，盘外壁用青花绘牵牛花，入窑高温烧成，再将黄釉施于青花纹饰之外，低温烘烧而成。黄釉青花始创于明，至清代仍十分流行。此盘青花浓重，有层次感，黄釉光亮，色调对比强烈，是清乾隆器中的佳品。

南京市博物馆藏

The plate has an everted mouth, a shallow curved belly, and a ring foot. The center is painted with nine peaches with morning glories intertwining around them; the patterns are in underglaze blue. The plate was first kilned in high temperature, then was coated with yellow glaze, and finally baked in low temperature. Yellow-glazed blue-and-white porcelain originated in the Ming Dynasty, and was still very popular in the Qing Dynasty. The dish is an outstanding masterpiece among those in Qianlong Reign of the Qing Dynasty, for its densely painted blue-and-white patterns with distinct layers, glossy yellow glaze, and the sharp contrast between colors.

Preserved in Nanjing Museum

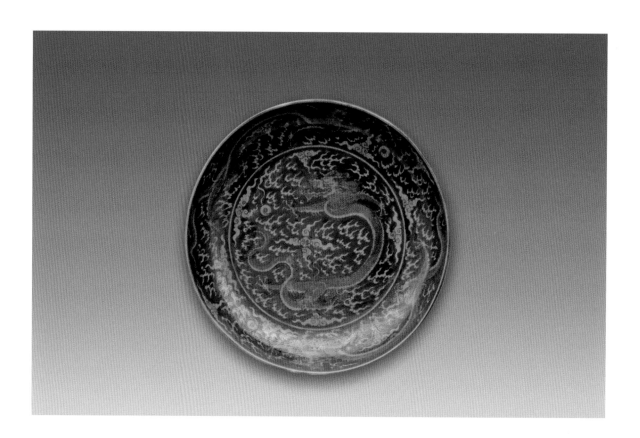

黑地绿龙纹盘

清

瓷质

口径 32 厘米，底径 22 厘米，通高 5.5 厘米

Plate Painted with Green Dragons Against Black Background

Qing Dynasty

Porcelain

Mouth Diameter 32 cm/ Bottom Diameter 22 cm/ Height 5.5 cm

侈口，浅弧腹，平底，矮圈足。盘心绘龙戏珠纹，隙地加云纹和火纹，内壁及外壁黑地绘二龙赶珠纹饰，近底边加莲瓣纹一周。器底施白釉，用青花绘双圈并书"大清康熙年制"六字两行楷书款。

南京市博物馆藏

The plate has a flared mouth, a shallow curved belly, a flat bottom, and a short ring foot. The center is patterned with a dragon playing with a pearl interspersed with cloud and fire patterns. The interior and exterior walls are painted with patterns of two dragons chasing a pearl against the black background; the lower part of the plate near the base is decorated with a circle of lotus petal patterns. The bottom is coated with white glaze and inscribed with six Chinese characters "Da Qing Kang Xi Nian Zhi" (made during Kangxi Reign of the Qing Dynasty) which are written in regular script in two lines and surrounded by blue-and-white double rings.
Preserved in Nanjing Museum

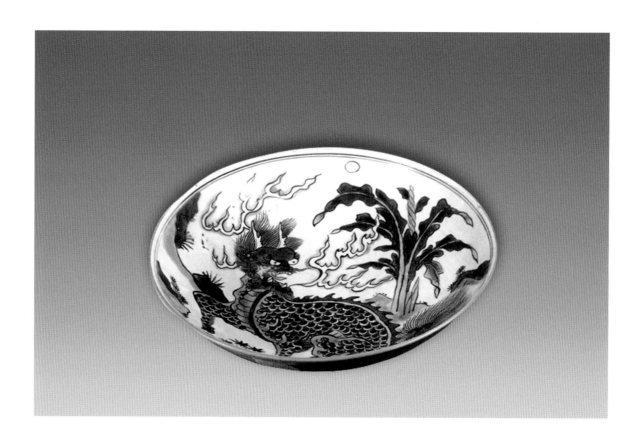

宫廷青花冰盘

清

瓷质

通高 8.2 厘米

Royal Blue-and-white Ice-plate

Qing Dynasty

Porcelain

Height 8.2 cm

敞口,圈足,内绘麒麟纹,圈足内有"玉堂佳口"
四字。为盛夏放冰用具,可防止食物变质或使
室内降温。

中国医史博物馆藏

The plate has an everted mouth and a ring foot
inscribed with Chinese characters "Yu Tang Jia
Kou" with kylin patterns inside. The plate was
used to keep ice in summer to prevent food from
decaying or to cool a room.

Preserved in China Medical History Museum

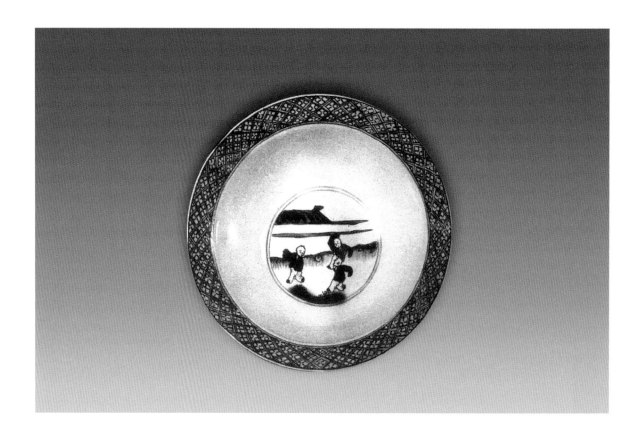

童子蹴鞠纹蒿花瓷盘

清

瓷质

口径 20.5 厘米

Porcelain Plate Painted with Netted Rhombus and Children Playing Cuju Ball

Qing Dynasty

Porcelain

Mouth Diameter 20.5 cm

瓷盘出自景德镇窑。广口，阔底，圈足。胎质细腻。器内上部饰以网状菱形纹，底部有三个童子做踢球游戏的画面，并以远景房屋和近景草地为衬饰。构图疏密有致，意趣盎然。

法国吉美国立亚洲艺术博物馆藏

The porcelain plate, which was made in Jingdezhen Kiln, has an everted mouth, a wide bottom, and a ring foot. Its pottery body is fine and smooth. The upper part is ornamented with netted rhombus patterns, and the center is painted with three children playing a cuju ball, with a house in the far distance and a grassland in the vicinity. The composition is well-conceived, displaying an amusing and vivid scene.

Preserved in Musée National des Arts Asiatiques-Guimet, France

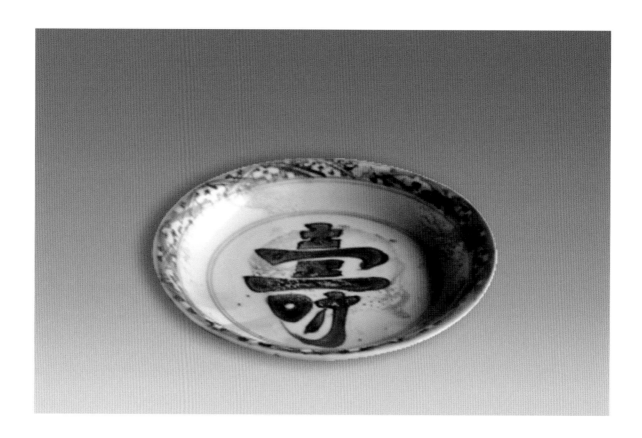

盘

清

瓷质

口径 13.5 厘米，通高 2.5 厘米

Plate

Qing Dynasty

Porcelain

Mouth Diameter 13.5 cm/ Height 2.5 cm

撇口，浅腹微斜，阔底，圈足。器内上部饰
以网格状花纹，盘内底有"寿"字，由民间
征集。

成都中医药大学中医药传统文化博物馆藏

The plate has an everted mouth, a short belly
that is slightly sloping, a wide bottom, and a
ring foot. The inner upper rim is decorated with
netlike patterns. There is a Chinese character
"Shou" (longevity) on its center. The plate was
collected from a private owner.

Preserved in the Museum of Medicine Preserved
in Museum of Traditional Chinese Medicine
Culture, Chengdu University of Traditional
Chinese Medicine

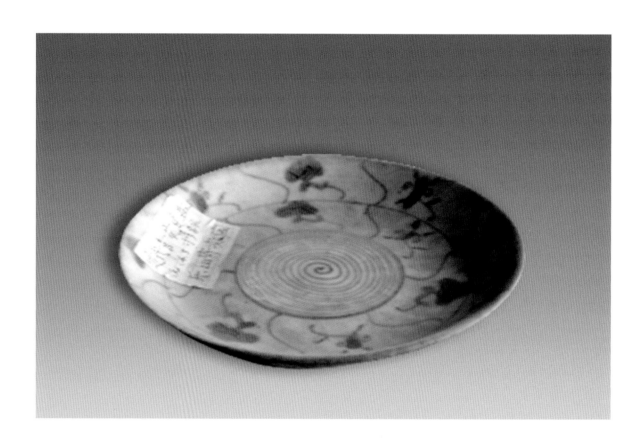

盘

清

瓷质

口径 15 厘米，通高 3 厘米

Plate

Qing Dynasty

Porcelain

Mouth Diameter 15 cm/ Height 3 cm

广口，阔底，圈足。内饰青花纹，盆底中心
饰顺时针旋转纹。由民间征集。

成都中医药大学中医药传统文化博物馆藏

The plate has a wide mouth, a broad bottom, and a ring foot. It is decorated with blue-and-white patterns on the inside and clockwise spiraling patterns in the center. The plate was collected from a private owner.

Preserved in Museum of Traditional Chinese Medicine Culture, Chengdu University of Traditional Chinese Medicine

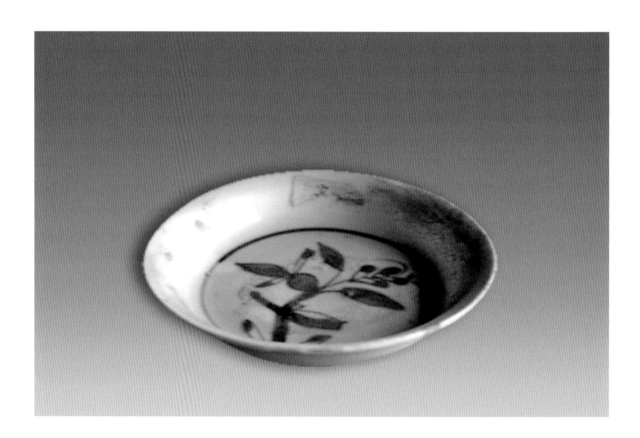

盘

清

瓷质

口径 10.5 厘米，通高 2 厘米

Plate

Qing Dynasty

Porcelain

Mouth Diameter 10.5 cm/ Height 2 cm

侈口，浅斜腹，阔底，圈足，底内饰花纹。

由民间征集。

　　成都中医药大学中医药传统文化博物馆藏

The plate has a flared mouth, a slightly sloping belly, a broad bottom, and a ring foot. It is decorated with flower patterns on the inside. The plate was collected from a private owner.

Preserved in Museum of Traditional Chinese Medicine Culture, Chengdu University of Traditional Chinese Medicine

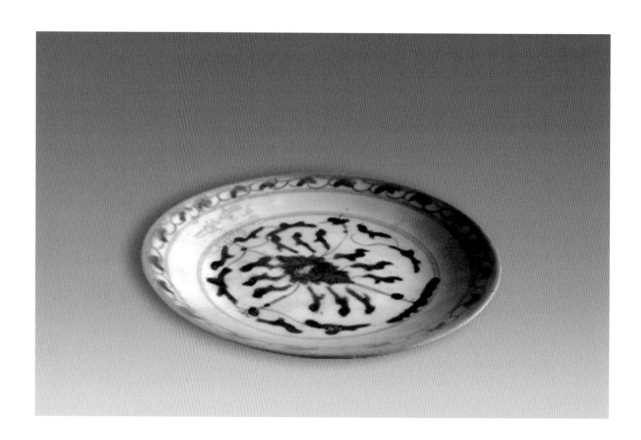

盘

清

瓷质

口径 18 厘米，通高 2.5 厘米

Plate

Qing Dynasty

Porcelain

Mouth Diameter 18 cm/ Height 2.5 cm

敞口，浅斜腹，阔底，圈足。青花纹饰。由民间征集。

成都中医药大学中医药传统文化博物馆藏

The plate with blue-and-white patterns has an everted mouth, a slightly sloping belly, a broad bottom, and a ring foot. It was collected from a private owner.

Preserved in Museum of Traditional Chinese Medicine Culture, Chengdu University of Traditional Chinese Medicine

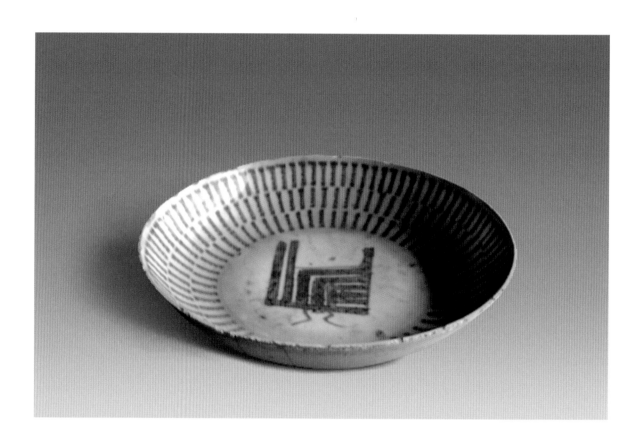

盘

清

瓷质

口径 19.5 厘米，通高 4 厘米

Plate

Qing Dynasty

Porcelain

Mouth Diameter 19.5 cm/ Height 4 cm

敞口，浅斜腹，阔底，圈足。青花纹饰。由民间征集。

成都中医药大学中医药传统文化博物馆藏

The dish with blue-and-white patterns has an everted mouth, a slightly sloping belly, a broad bottom, and a ring foot. It was collected from a private owner.

Preserved in Museum of Traditional Chinese Medicine Culture, Chengdu University of Traditional Chinese Medicine

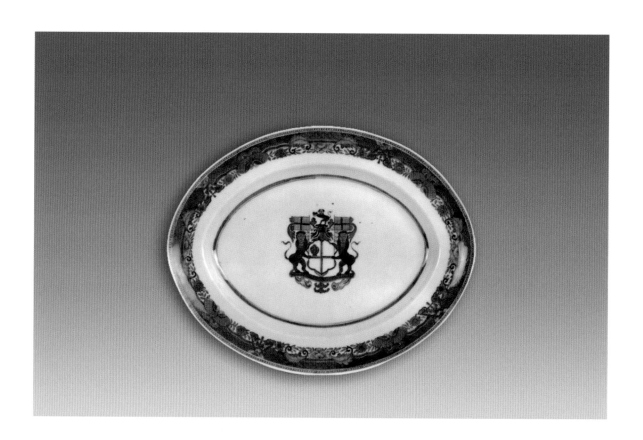

青花盘

清

瓷质

口径 30.4 厘米

盘形椭圆折腹，圈足。

沙巴治藏

Blue-and-white Plate

Qing Dynasty

Porcelain

Mouth Diameter 30.4 cm

The oblate plate has a folded belly and a ring foot.

Collected by António Sapage

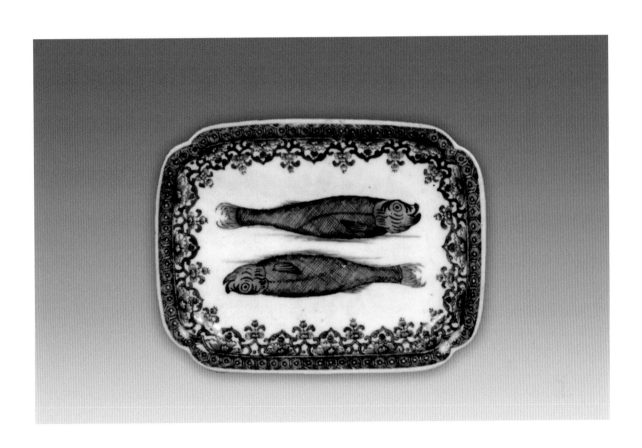

青花鱼纹盘

清

瓷质

口径 24 厘米

长方形。花瓣口，内饰缠枝花纹一周，盆底饰青

花鱼纹。

沙巴治藏

Blue-and-white Plate Patterned with Fish

Qing Dynasty

Porcelain

Mouth Diameter 24 cm

The rectangular plate has a petal-shaped mouth and intertwining branches around its inner wall and blue-and-white patterns at the bottom.

Collected by António Sapage

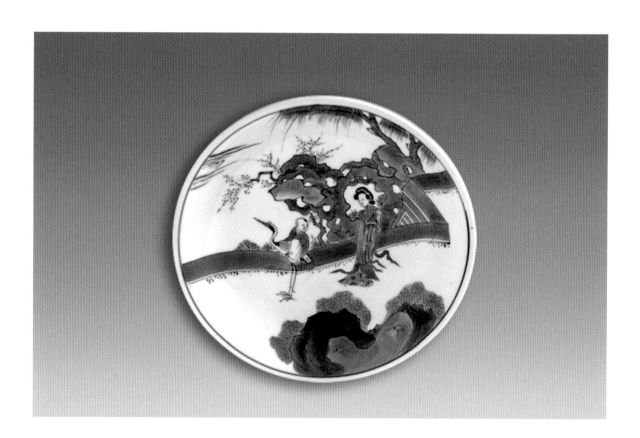

青花妇婴戏鹤图盘

清

瓷质

口径 15.8 厘米，底径 7 厘米

Blue-and-white Plate with Scene of Woman and Child Playing with Crane

Qing Dynasty

Porcelain

Mouth Diameter 15.8 cm/ Bottom Diameter 7 cm

敞口，浅腹，圈足。盘内绘一小孩骑在一鹤
背上，背后站着一妇女相望，周围衬假山石、
杨柳、梅花等纹饰，青花鲜艳，白釉莹润，
是康熙青花上乘之作。

李鸿基藏

The plate has an everted mouth, a shallow
belly, and a ring foot. The painting on the plate
portrays a child riding on a crane and in the
rear a lady is watching them. The figures are
surrounded by patterns of rockeries, willows
and plum blossoms. The plate was one of the
best during Kangxi Reign of the Qing Dynasty
for its brilliant blue-and-white patterns and
glossy white glaze.

Collected by Li Hongji

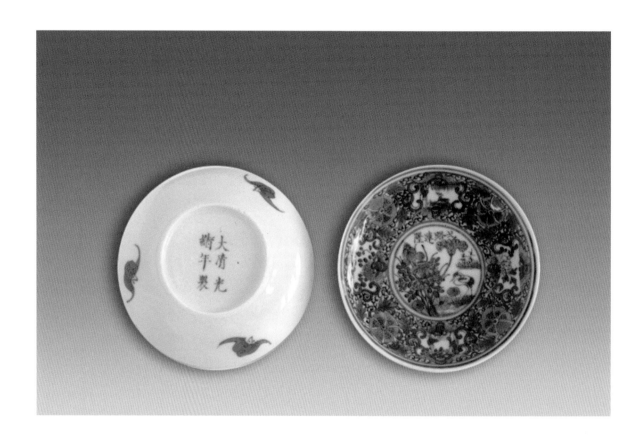

青花花鸟纹盘（一对）

清

瓷质

口径 12 厘米

A Pair of Blue-and-white Plates Patterned with Flowers and Birds

Qing Dynasty

Porcelain

Mouth Diameter 12 cm

敞口，浅腹，圈足。内绘荷花、鹭鸟纹，书写"一路连升"四字。外壁绘三只蝙蝠，底书写"大清光绪年制"六字楷书款。青花呈色鲜艳，是光绪年间民间佳作。

刘建业藏

The dish has an everted mouth, a shallow belly, and a ring foot. Its center is decorated with lotuses, an egret, and Chinese inscriptions "Yi Lu Lian Sheng" (getting promoted constantly). The exterior wall is decorated with three bats. The bottom is inscribed with six words "Da Qing Guang Xu Nian Zhi" (made during Guangxu Reign of the Qing Dynasty) in regular script. The plate, with bright and vivid patterns, is one of the best made by folk workmen during Guangxu Reign of the Qing Dynasty.

Collected by Liu Jianye

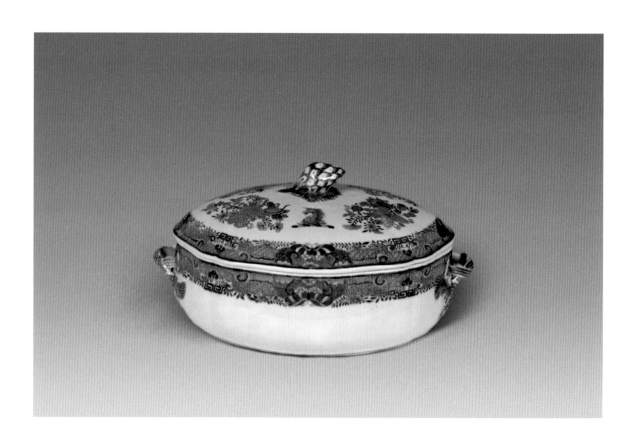

青花带盖盘

清

瓷质

口径 32 厘米

Blue-and-white Plate with Lid

Qing Dynasty

Porcelain

Mouth Diameter 32 cm

圆形，两侧附编织纽带形为耳。盘边缘和盖
缘绘缠枝花纹，盖面绘折枝花卉，还饰有英
国比雅利家族纹章。

沙巴治藏

The round plate has a pair of handles shaped
like weaved links on both sides. The rims of the
plate and its lid are decorated with intertwining
flower patterns. The lid surface is painted with
plucked branches and the insignia of a British
family.

Collected by António Sapage

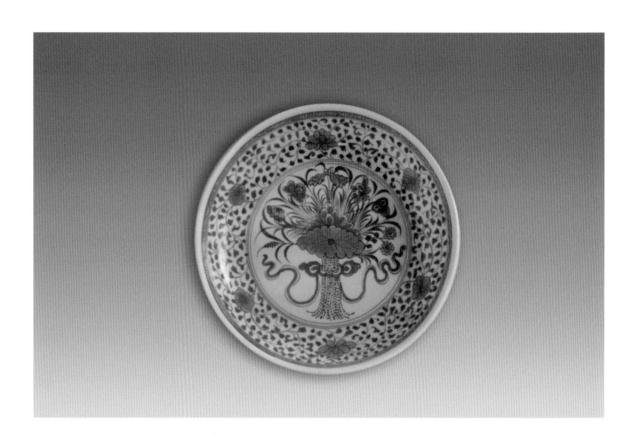

青花束莲纹盘

清

瓷质

口径 25.8 厘米

Blue-and-white Plate with Lotus Patterns

Qing Dynasty

Porcelain

Mouth Diameter 25.8 cm

敞口，弧形腹，圈足。外壁口沿画弦纹一道，内壁上下画弦纹，内绘缠枝花卉，盘心饰一束莲花，青花鲜艳。施白釉稍泛青色，胎坚洁，为雍正年间民窑的产品。

黄东海藏

The plate has an everted mouth, a curved belly, and a ring foot. The exterior wall rim is decorated with a circle of bowstring patterns and the interior wall is decorated with, two circles of bowstring patterns with intertwining flower patterns between them. In the center of the plate there is a lotus. The dish, with a solid and clean pottery body, is coated with white glaze with a tinge of cyan. It was made in a non-governmental kiln during Yongzheng Reign of the Qing Dynasty.

Collected by Huang Donghai

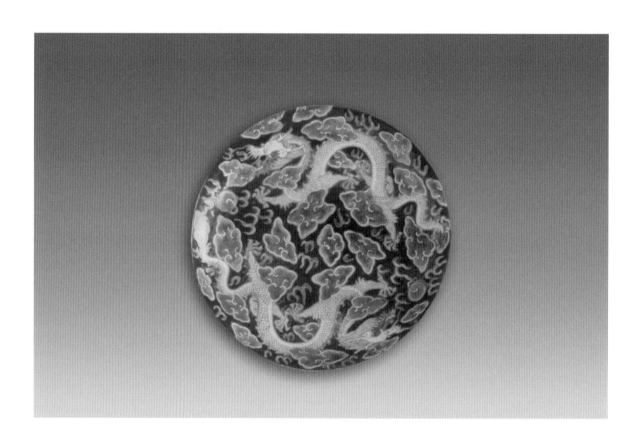

蓝地红龙纹盘

清

瓷质

口径 15 厘米

Plate Painted with Red Dragons Against Blue Background

Qing Dynasty

Porcelain

Mouth Diameter 15 cm

敞口，浅腹，圈足。盘内施蓝地彩，上绘红彩云龙纹，色彩华贵艳丽。底书写"大清光绪年制"六字青花楷书款。

梁权藏

The plate has an everted mouth, a shallow belly, and a ring foot. On its interior wall there are two red-glazed dragons amid clouds of the same color against the blue background. The colors are gorgeous. The bottom is inscribed with six blue-and white words "Da Qing Guang Xu Nian Zhi" (made during Guangxu Reign the the Qing Dynasty) in regular script.

Collected by Liang Quan

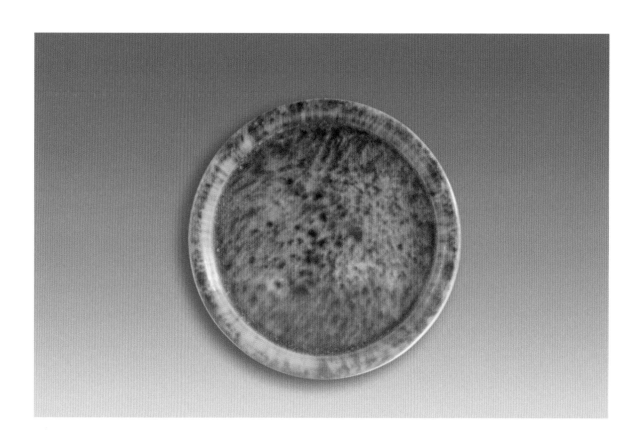

石湾窑洒蓝釉托盘

清

瓷质

口径 30 厘米，底径 27 厘米，通高 3 厘米

Snowflake Blue-glazed Saucer, Shiwan Kiln

Qing Dynasty

Porcelain

Mouth Diameter 30 cm/ Bottom Diameter 27 cm/ Height 3 cm

板缘，浅腹，平底。施釉厚润，蓝白相间。石湾窑是仿宋钧窑，以造型和釉色取胜。该盘造型古拙，釉色奇丽，是石湾窑的佳品。

麦森炽藏

The saucer has a semi-cylinderical rim, a shallow belly, and a flat bottom. The thickly and smoothly glazed saucer displays blue and white flecks spaced in between. Shiwan Kiln-made ceramics, as a copy of Jun Kiln ware made in the Song Dynasty, stands out among the same kind for their modelling and glaze. The unsophisticatedly shaped saucer, with unique and marvelous glaze, is an outstanding one among those made in Shiwan Kiln.

Collected by Mai Senchi

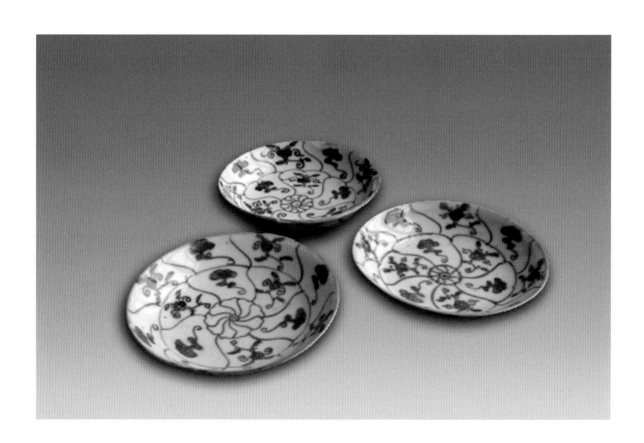

瓷碟

清

瓷质

口径 10.8 厘米，高 2.7 厘米

Porcelain Dishes

Qing Dynasty

Porcelain

Mouth Diameter 10.8 cm/ Height 2.7 cm

园形兰花小碟。敞口，浅斜腹，圈足，内饰。

江苏省中医药博物馆藏

Each of the dishes covered with orchid patterns on the inside has an everted mouth, a slightly sloping belly, and a ring foot.

Preserved by Jiangsu Museum of Traditional Chinese Medicine

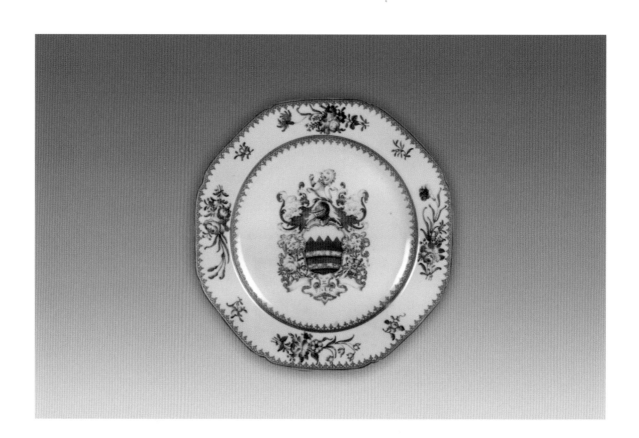

广彩碟

清

瓷质

口径 22 厘米

Guangzhou Overglaze Porcelain Dish

Qing Dynasty

Porcelain

Mouth Diameter 22 cm

析沿，浅圆底，盘沿饰4组花卉，内绘有Hare家族的徽章。

沙巴治藏

The dish has a folded rim and a round shallow bottom. The rim is decorated with four groups of flower patterns. There is an insignia of Hare's Family in the center of the dish.

Collected by António Sapage

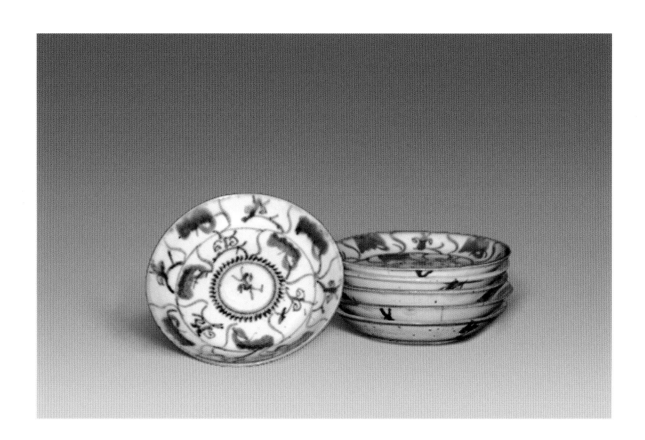

蓝花瓷碟

清

瓷质

口径 14 厘米，底径 8.5 厘米，通高 2.5 厘米，重 160 克

Blue-and-white Porcelain Dishes Painted with Floral Motifs

Qing Dynasty

Porcelain

Mouth Diameter 14 cm/ Bottom Diameter 8.5 cm/ Height 2.5 cm/ Weight 160 g

敞口，斜腹，圈足。青花，底部有"无""太"
等图案。食器。陕西省西安市八仙庵征集，
2001 年 9 月入藏，有裂痕。

陕西医史博物馆藏

The blue-and-white dishes have wide and slightly
everted rim, an inclined belly, and a ring feet. The
bottom is inscribed with such Chinese characters
as " 无 " (Wu) and " 太 " (Tai) . The dishes with
cracks were used as dining utensils. The artifacts
were collected from the Temple of the Eight
Immortals in Xi'an, Shaanxi Province, and came
into the museum's collection in September 2011.
Preserved in Shaanxi Museum of Medical History

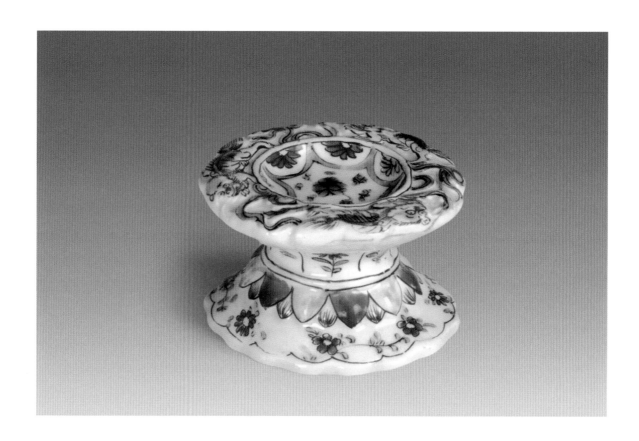

五彩高足花碟

清

瓷质

通高 8.3 厘米

Five-color High-footed Dish Painted with Floral Motifs

Qing Dynasty

Porcelain

Height 8.3 cm

椭圆形口，树根形底坐，梅花图。生活用具。
陕西省澄城县征集。有裂印。

陕西医史博物馆藏

The cup, which was for daily use, has an oval
mouth, a tree root-shaped stand, a carved and
relief design of plum blossoms on one side, and
some crackles. It was collected from Chengcheng
County, Shaanxi Province.

Preserved in Shaanxi Museum of Medical History

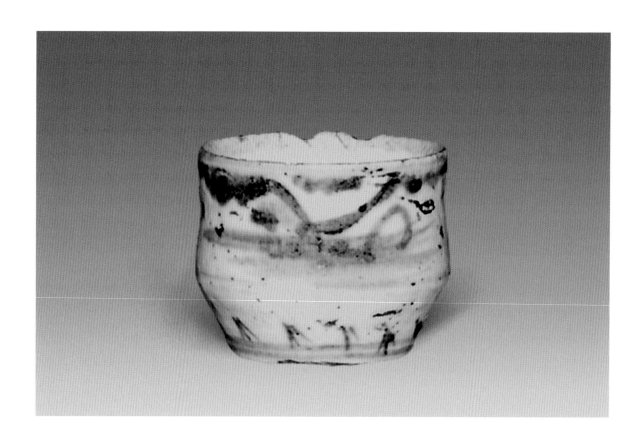

小瓷杯

清

瓷质

口径 6.5 厘米，底径 5 厘米，通高 5.5 厘米，重 500 克

直口，折腹，圈足，有"小兰花"图案。生活用器，口沿有小残损。

陕西医史博物馆藏

Small Porcelain Cup

Qing Dynasty

Porcelain

Mouth diameter 6.5 cm/ Bottom diameter 5 cm/ Height 5.5 cm/ Weight 500 g

The cup, which was for daily use, has a vertical mouth, an inclined belly, and a foot ring. It is decorated with scrolled iris patterns. The rim is slightly damaged.

Preserved in Shaanxi Museum of Medical History

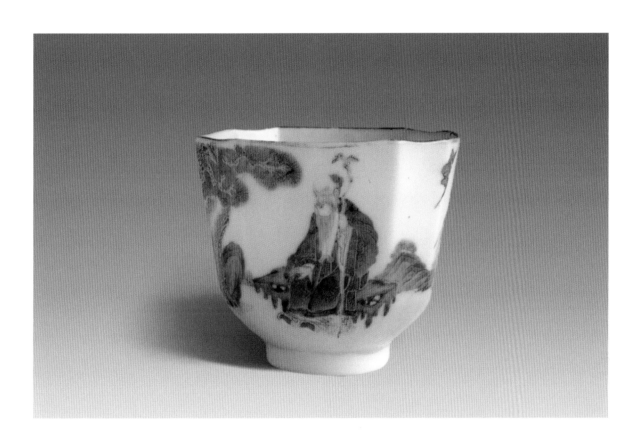

粉彩八角形杯

清

瓷质

口径 7.8 厘米，底径 3.9 厘米，通高 7 厘米

杯身绘一老寿星，以及古松、飞蝠等纹饰。

邝顺佳藏

Octagonal Cup in Famille Rose

Qing Dynasty

Porcelain

Mouth Diameter 7.8 cm/ Bottom Diameter 3.9 cm/ Height 7 cm

The principal motifs are a god of longevity, an old pine tree, and a flying bat in blue, yellow and greenish palette enamel on the exterior.

Collected by Kuang Shunjia

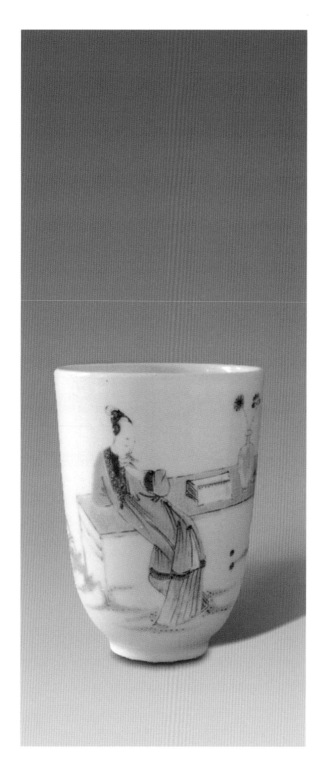

粉彩仕女马铃形杯

清

瓷质

通高 9 厘米

Sleigh Bell-shaped Famille Rose Cup Painted with a Beautiful Lady

Qing Dynasty

Porcelain

Height 9 cm

侈口，往下渐收，高身，圈足，似一仰马铃。里外施白釉。外壁一头梳高髻的女子倚桌而立，桌上放一梳妆盒和一插着鲜花的花瓶。画面简洁疏朗，却很雅致。为康熙时一种常见的器型。

高丰藏

Looking like an upright sleigh bell, the cup has a flared mouth, deep sides with tapered lower part, and a ring foot. The cup is coated with white glaze all over. On the exterior wall of the cup there is a beautiful lady (with a high bun) leaning against a table, on which there are a dressing case and a vase with flowers in it. Those painted, though concise and sparse, are elegant. The model of the cup was common during Kangxi Period of the Qing Dynasty.

Collected by Gao Feng

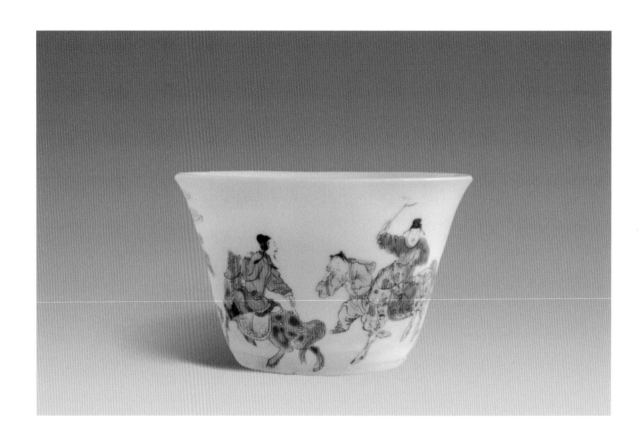

粉彩人马纹杯

清

瓷质

口径 9 厘米

Famille Rose Cup Painted with Figures and Horses

Qing Dynasty

Porcelain

Mouth Diameter 9 cm

撇口，口往下渐收，卧足。外壁彩绘两人各骑一匹马在奔跑着，旁有一书童背书相随。色彩莹润鲜艳。该藏是雍正粉彩代表作。

李牧之藏

The cup has an everted mouth, a tapered body, and a concave foot. On the exterior wall there are two men riding on horses, followed by a page boy carrying books, The glaze is glossy and brilliant. The cup was a representative famille rose work in Yongzheng Reign of the Qing Dynasty.

Collected by Li Muzhi

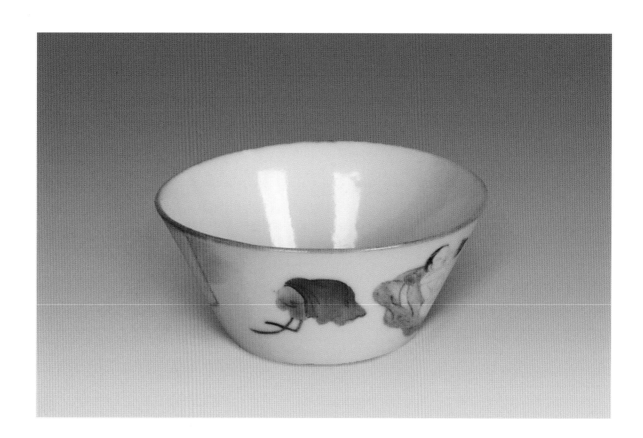

人物套杯

清

瓷质

口径 8.5 厘米，底径 4.8 厘米，通高 4 厘米

Cup (of a Set) Painted with Figures

Qing Dynasty

Porcelain

Mouth Diameter 8.5 cm/ Bottom Diameter 4.8 cm/ Height 4 cm

碗形。敞口，平底，圈足。该组套杯粉彩釉，
釉色润泽光洁，绘各式春宫图，工艺精细。
为盛器。1957 年入藏，保存完好。

中华医学会 / 上海中医药大学医史博物馆

The bowl-like cup has an everted mouth, a
flat bottom, and a ring foot. On the exterior
wall there is a pornographic picture in
famille rose palette enamel, which is glossy
and clean. The exquisite cup was collected
by the museum in 1957 and is still in good
condition.
Preserved in Chinese Medical Association/
Museum of Chinese Medicine, Shanghai
University of Traditional Chinese Medicine

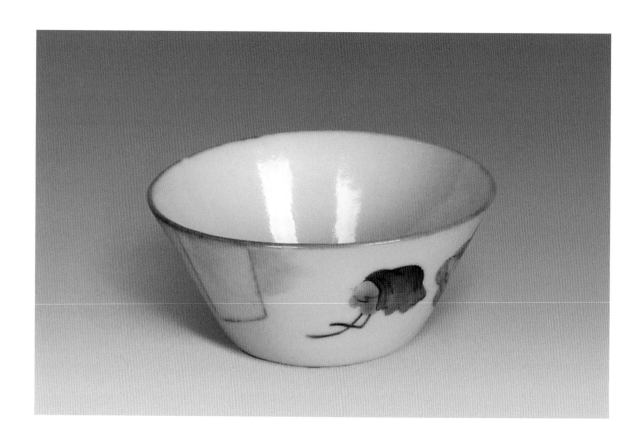

人物套杯

清

瓷质

口径 7.1 厘米，底径 4.2 厘米，通高 2.95 厘米

Cup (of a Set) Painted with Figures

Qing Dynasty

Porcelain

Mouth Diameter 7.1 cm/ Bottom Diameter 4.2 cm/ Height 2.95 cm

碗形。敞口，平底，圈足。该组套杯粉彩釉，
釉色润泽光洁，绘各式春宫图，工艺精细。
为盛器。1957 年入藏，保存完好。

中华医学会 / 上海中医药大学医史博物馆

The bowl-like cup has an everted mouth, a
flat bottom, and a ring foot. On the exterior
wall there is a pornographic picture in
famille rose palette enamel, which is glossy
and clean. The exquisite cup was collected
by the museum in 1957 and is still in good
condition.

Preserved in Chinese Medical Association/
Museum of Chinese Medicine, Shanghai
University of Traditional Chinese Medicine

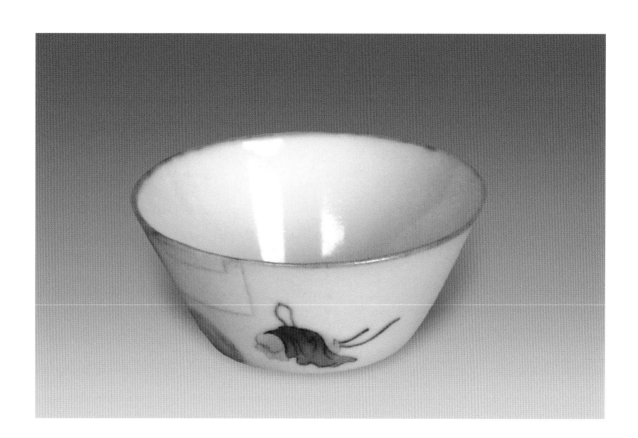

人物套杯

清

瓷质

口径 6.6 厘米，底径 3.7 厘米，通高 2.55 厘米

Cup (of a Set) Painted with Figures

Qing Dynasty

Porcelain

Mouth Diameter 6.6 cm/ Bottom Diameter 3.7 cm/ Height 2.55 cm

碗形。敞口，平底，圈足。该组套杯粉彩釉，
釉色润泽光洁，绘各式春宫图，工艺精细。
为盛器。1957 年入藏，保存完好。

中华医学会 / 上海中医药大学医史博物馆

The bowl-like cup has an everted mouth, a
flat bottom, and a ring foot. On the exterior
wall there is a pornographic picture in famille
rose palette enamel, which is glossy and
clean. The exquisite cup was collected by
the museum in 1957 and is still in good
condition.

Preserved in Chinese Medical Association/
Museum of Chinese Medicine, Shanghai
University of Traditional Chinese Medicine

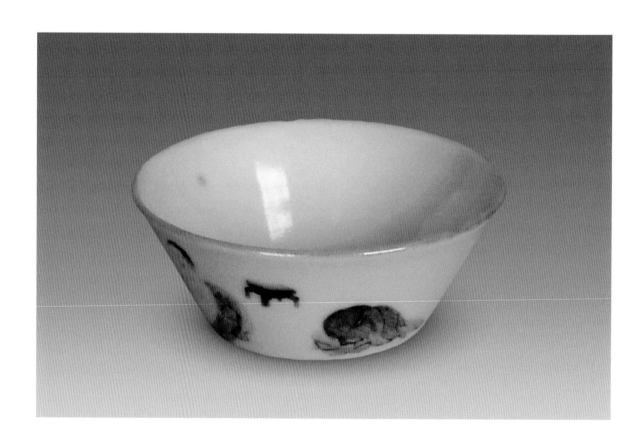

人物套杯

清

瓷质

口径 6.1 厘米，底径 3.5 厘米，通高 2.4 厘米

Cup (of a Set) Painted with Figures

Qing Dynasty

Porcelain

Mouth Diameter 6.1 cm/ Bottom Diameter 3.5 cm/ Height 2.4 cm

碗形。敞口，平底，圈足。该组套杯粉彩釉，

釉色润泽光洁，绘各式春宫图，工艺精细。

为盛器。1957 年入藏，保存完好。

中华医学会 / 上海中医药大学医史博物馆

The bowl-like cup has an everted mouth, a
flat bottom, and a ring foot. On the exterior
wall there is a pornographic picture in famille
rose palette enamel, which is glossy and
clean. The exquisite cup was collected by
the museum in 1957 and is still in good
condition.

Preserved in Chinese Medical Association/
Museum of Chinese Medicine, Shanghai
University of Traditional Chinese Medicine

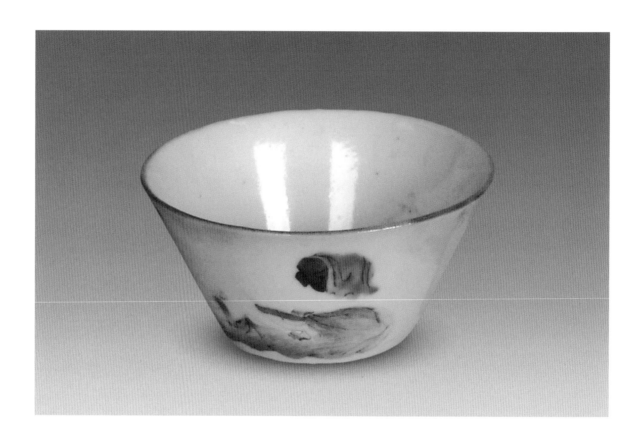

人物套杯

清

瓷质

口径 7.9 厘米，底径 4.3 厘米，通高 3.6 厘米

Cup (of a Set) Painted with Figures

Qing Dynasty

Porcelain

Mouth Diameter 7.9 cm/ Bottom Diameter 4.3 cm/ Height 3.6 cm

碗形。敞口，平底，圈足。该组套杯粉彩釉，
釉色润泽光洁，绘各式春宫图，工艺精细。
为盛器。1957 年入藏，保存完好。

中华医学会 / 上海中医药大学医史博物馆

The bowl-like cup has an everted mouth, a
flat bottom, and a ring foot. On the exterior
wall there is a pornographic picture in famille
rose palette enamel, which is glossy and
clean. The exquisite cup was collected by
the museum in 1957 and is still in good
condition.

Preserved in Chinese Medical Association/
Museum of Chinese Medicine, Shanghai
University of Traditional Chinese Medicine

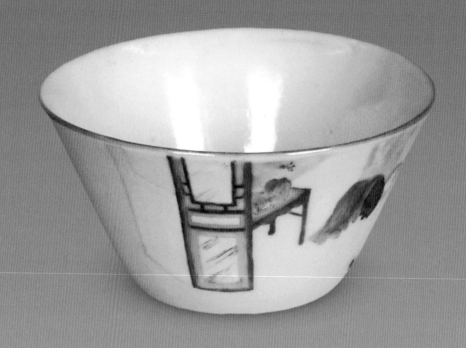

人物套杯

清

瓷质

口径 9.5 厘米，底径 5.2 厘米，通高 4.4 厘米

Cup (of a Set) Painted with Figures

Qing Dynasty

Porcelain

Mouth Diameter 9.5 cm/ Bottom Diameter 5.2 cm/ Height 4.4 cm

碗形。敞口，平底，圈足。该组套杯粉彩釉，
釉色润泽光洁，绘各式春宫图，工艺精细。
为盛器。1957 年入藏，保存完好。

中华医学会 / 上海中医药大学医史博物馆

The bowl-like cup has an everted mouth, a
flat bottom, and a ring foot. On the exterior
wall there is a pornographic picture in famille
rose palette enamel, which is glossy and
clean. The exquisite cup was collected by
the museum in 1957 and is still in good
condition.

Preserved in Chinese Medical Association/
Museum of Chinese Medicine, Shanghai
University of Traditional Chinese Medicine

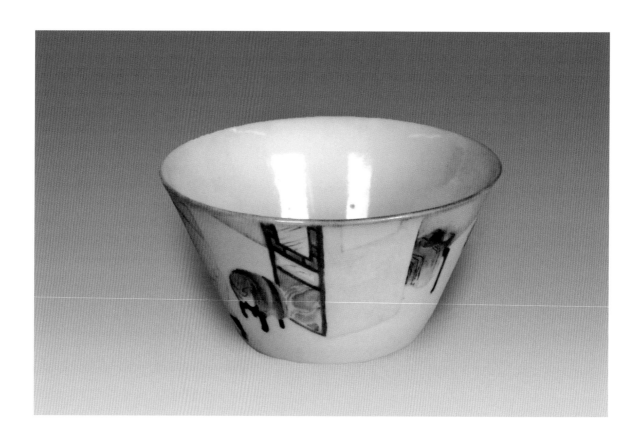

人物套杯

清

瓷质

口径 9.5 厘米，底径 5.2 厘米，通高 4.4 厘米

Cup (of a Set) Painted with Figures

Qing Dynasty

Porcelain

Mouth Diameter 9.5 cm/ Bottom Diameter 5.2 cm/ Height 4.4 cm

碗形。敞口，平底，圈足。该组套杯粉彩釉，釉色润泽光洁，绘各式春宫图，工艺精细。为盛器。1957 年入藏，保存完好。

中华医学会 / 上海中医药大学医史博物馆

The bowl-like cup has an everted mouth, a flat bottom, and a ring foot. On the exterior wall there is a pornographic picture in famille rose palette enamel, which is glossy and clean. The exquisite cup was collected by the museum in 1957 and is still in good condition.

Preserved in Chinese Medical Association/ Museum of Chinese Medicine, Shanghai University of Traditional Chinese Medicine

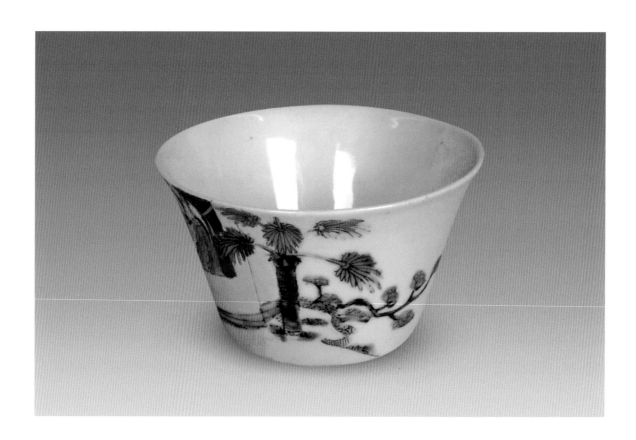

人物套杯

清

瓷质

口径 10.2 厘米，底径 5.5 厘米，通高 5.1 厘米

Cup (of a Set) Painted with Figures

Qing Dynasty

Porcelain

Mouth Diameter 10.2 cm/ Bottom Diameter 5.5 cm/ Height 5.1 cm

碗形。敞口，平底，圈足。该组套杯粉彩釉，
釉色润泽光洁，绘各式春宫图，工艺精细。
为盛器。1957 年入藏，保存完好。

中华医学会 / 上海中医药大学医史博物馆

The bowl-like cup has an everted mouth, a
flat bottom, and a ring foot. On the exterior
wall there is a pornographic picture in famille
rose palette enamel, which is glossy and
clean. The exquisite cup was collected by
the museum in 1957 and is still in good
condition.

Preserved in Chinese Medical Association/
Museum of Chinese Medicine, Shanghai
University of Traditional Chinese Medicine

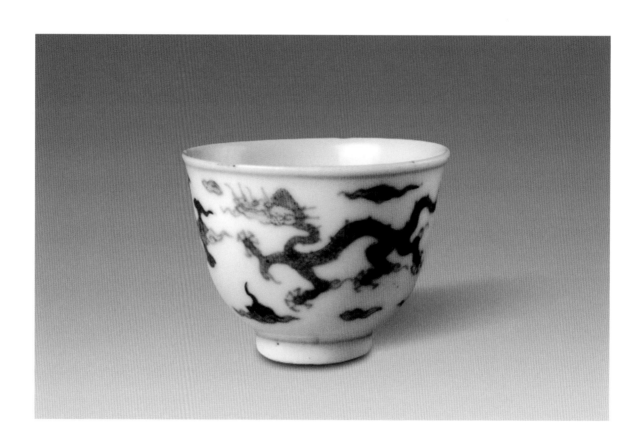

斗彩云龙纹杯

清

瓷质

口径 9 厘米

Doucai Cup with Cloud and Dragon Motifs

Qing Dynasty

Porcelain

Mouth Diameter 9 cm

造型为敞口，往下渐收，小圈足，胎薄。腹部主题纹饰绘云龙如意纹，施白釉甚匀净。

杜灿佳藏

The cup has an everted mouth, a tapered body, and a small foot ring. It is covered with thin and evenly-distributed white glaze and painted with auspicious cloud and dragon motifs on the exterior.

Collected by Du Canjia

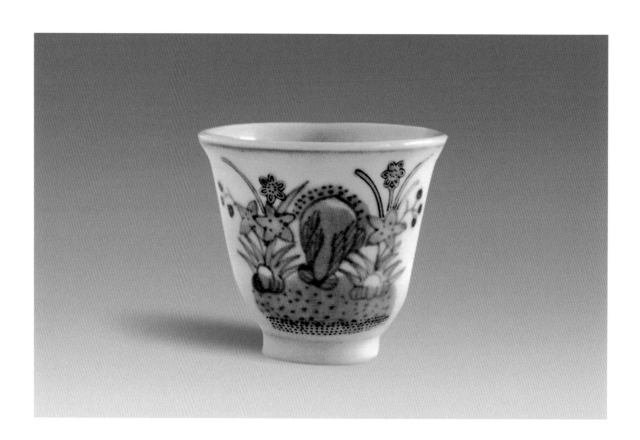

斗彩花卉小杯

清

瓷质

口径 4.7 厘米，通高 5.5 厘米

Small Doucai Cup Painted with Floral Motifs

Qing Dynasty

Porcelain

Mouth Diameter 4.7 cm/ Height 5.5 cm

敞口稍外撇，至足渐收，深腹圈足。口沿处画一青花弦纹，腹部以青花勾画山石、花卉枝叶的轮廓，然后以红、黄、绿等色彩绘。里外施白釉，小巧玲珑，颇为雅玩，底有"大清光绪年制"六字楷书青花款。

梁权藏

The cup, which is coated with white glaze all over, has a slightly everted mouth, a deep belly with tapered lower part, and a ring foot. The mouth rim is decorated with blue-and-white bowstring designs. On the exterior there are rockeries and flowers with branches and leaves glazed in red, yellow and green, which are outlined in underglaze blue. The bottom of the cup is inscribed with Chinese words "Da Qing Guang Xu Nian Zhi" (made during Guangxu Reign of the Qing Dynasty) in regular script and underglaze blue. The cup is bijou and elegant.
Collected by Liang Quan

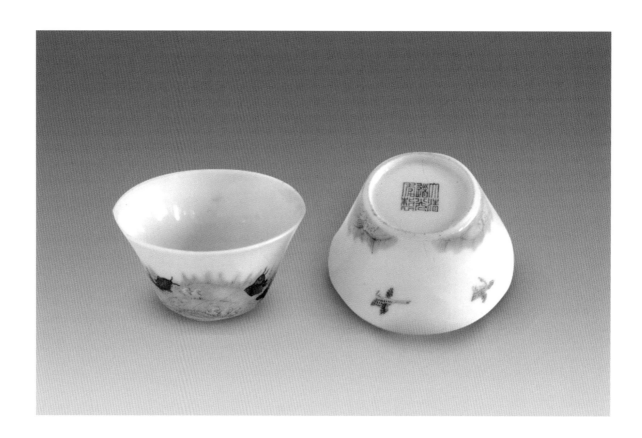

红绿彩鱼戏水纹马蹄形杯

清

瓷质

口径 11 厘米

Hoof-shaped Cup with Scene of Red Fish Frolicking in Green Water

Qing Dynasty

Porcelain

Mouth Diameter 11 cm

敞口，沿稍外折，矮圈足。腹部绘绿彩海水红彩鱼儿戏水纹，红彩鲜艳，画面十分生动。

杜灿佳藏

The cup has a wide and slightly everted mouth and a short ring foot. On the exterior wall some red fish painted with bright red glaze are frolicking in green water. The scene is very vivid.

Collected by Du Canjia

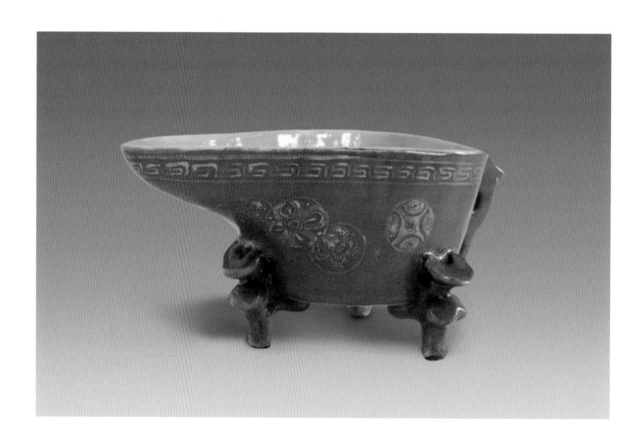

珊瑚红描金三足杯

清

瓷质

前后口径 4.8 厘米，左右口径 9.8 厘米，前后底径 4 厘米，左右底径 4.5 厘米，通高 5.1 厘米

Triple-footed Cup in Coral Red Glaze and with Golden Ball Motifs

Qing Dynasty

Porcelain

Mouth Diameter 4.8 cm by 9.8 cm/ Bottom Diameter 4 cm by 4.5 cm/ Height 5.1 cm

整个杯似一只倒放的古代中国妇女包裹的小脚，脚底朝天为杯口，十分形象。杯的底足用三棵磨菇支撑，外施珊瑚红釉，描金皮球花纹饰，内施青绿釉。杯执扁条状。这件作品造型新颖，艺术性较高。

李牧之藏

The cup resembles an inverted tiny bound foot of a lady in ancient China. The bound foot points upwards as the mouth of the cup. The cup is supported by three mushroom-shaped feet and has a strip-shaped handle. Its coral red-glazed exterior is decorated with golden ball motifs. The interior is coated with bean green glaze. The cup has ingenious modelling and high artistic value.

Collected by Li Muzhi

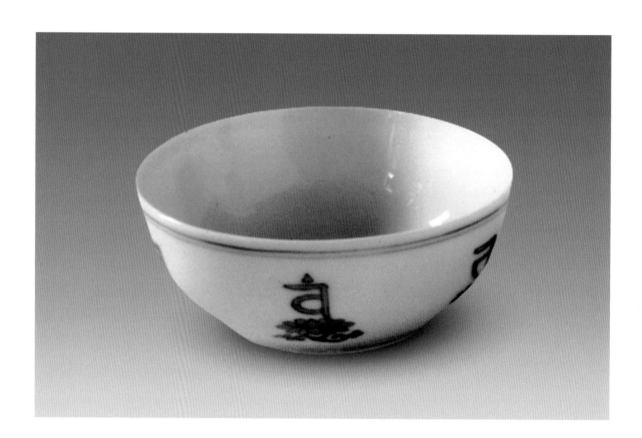

青花梵文杯

清

瓷质

口径 6.3 厘米

Blue-and-white Cup Painted with Sanskrit Characters

Qing Dynasty

Porcelain

Mouth Diameter 6.3 cm

敛口，鼓腹，圈足。口外沿画双弦纹，近足
处亦画弦纹一道，腹间以折枝花托梵文做装
饰，六个不同的梵文和花朵匀称地分布在小
杯周围。里外施白釉，细润而莹亮。圈足内
青花双方框，内两行直书"大清雍正年制"
楷书款，字体工整秀美，为雍正官窑作品。

高丰藏

The cup has a contracted mouth, a bulged
belly, and a foot ring. Its interior and exterior
are coated with white glaze, which is shiny
and fine. There are two bowstring designs near
the mouth rim and another bowstring design
near the foot. The body is decorated with six
different Sanskrit characters supported by six
plucked flowers spaced evenly. The foot is
inscribed with six neat and graceful Chinese
words in regular script "Da Qing Yong Zheng
Nian Zhi" (made during Yongzheng Reign of
the Qing Dynasty) arranged in two lines in
underglaze-blue double frames.

Collected by Gao Feng

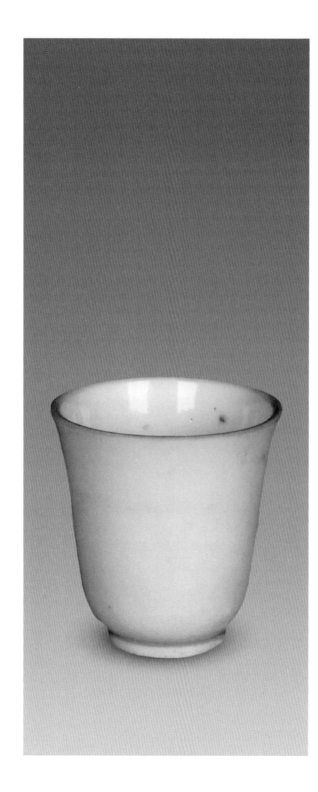

茶杯

清

瓷质

口外径 7.1 厘米，底径 3.8 厘米，通高 7.1 厘米

Tea Cup

Qing Dynasty

Porcelain

Mouth Outer Diameter 7.1 cm/ Bottom Diameter

3.8 cm/ Height 7.1 cm

杯形。该藏通身施白釉，敞口圈足无款，

工艺较好。为茶具。1956 年入藏，保存

基本完好。

中华医学会 / 上海中医药大学医史博物馆

The tea cup, which is coated with white glaze
all over, has an everted mouth and a foot
ring but no inscription. The delicate cup
was collected by the museum in 1956 and is
basically in good condition.

Preserved in Chinese Medical Association/
Museum of Chinese Medicine, Shanghai
University of Traditional Chinese Medicine

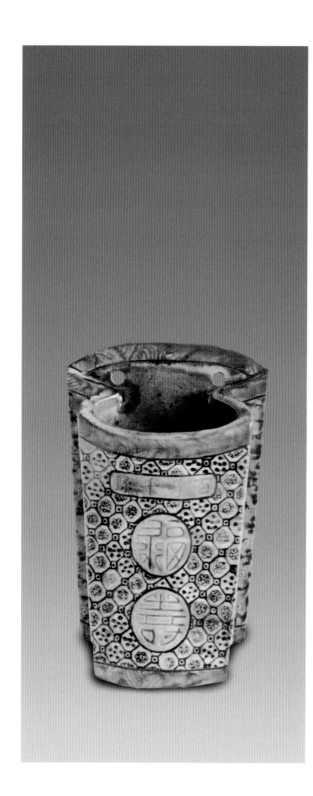

石湾窑筷子筒

清

瓷质

宽 15 厘米，通高 23.2 厘米

Chopsticks Container of Shiwan Kiln

Qing Dynasty

Porcelain

Width 15 cm/ Height 23.2 cm

筷子筒虽是日常生活用品，但此物造型奇特，以书卷的造型表现别有一番情趣。外饰以绿釉暗花，内以白地黑花为纹饰，中间刻有福寿篆书图案，设计颇费一番用心。

许荣坤藏

Despite its triviality as an article for daily use, this chopsticks container is peculiarly shaped: it is like a book volume. The upper and lower rims are decorated with indistinct green-glazed floral patterns. The surface is inscribed with Chinese words "Fu" (good fortune) and "Shou" (longevity) in seal script interspersed with black flowers against the white background, all of which show elaborate design.

Collected by Xu Rongkun

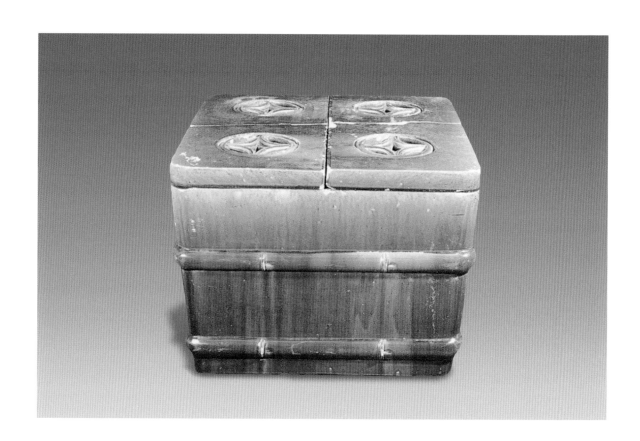

宫廷藏冰箱

清

琉璃质

上、下边长分别为 46.5 厘米、42.5 厘米，通高 24 厘米

Imperial Ice-box

Qing Dynasty

Glass

Upper Length 46.5 cm/ Lower Length 42.5 cm/ Height 24 cm

直口，平沿，口大底小呈斗形。箱外绕竹节
纹突起一周，盖分两块，各有两个钱孔散发
冷气。藏冰器皿，用于冷藏或调节室温。

中国医史博物馆藏

The glazed ice-box has a vertical mouth, a flat
rim, and a funnel-like shape with the mouth
bigger than the bottom. Protruding bamboo
joint designs surround the ice-box in a circle.
The lid has two segments, either of which has
two holes like a coin for emitting cold air. The
ice-box was used to refrigerate or adjust room
temperature.

Preserved in China Medical History Museum

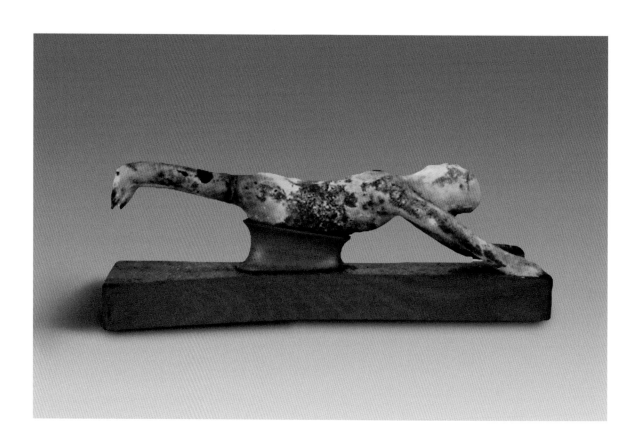

唐游泳俑（复制品）

清

陶质

宽 8.6 厘米，通高 6.8 厘米

Tang Swimming Figurine (Imitation)

Qing Dynasty

Pottery

Width 8.6 cm/ Height 6.8 cm

明器。该藏为清代复制唐代陶俑，灰黑色，

人物作游泳状，为古代健身运动文物。

1955 年入藏，保存基本完好 。

中华医学会 / 上海中医药大学医史博物馆

The swimming figurine, a burial object, was
copied in the Qing Dynasty from a model
made in the Tang Dynasty. The grayish black
swimming figurine is one of the relics that
depict ancient body-building exercises. It
was collected by the museum in 1955 and is
basically well preserved.

Preserved in Chinese Medical Association/
Museum of Chinese Medicine, Shanghai
University of Traditional Chinese Medicine

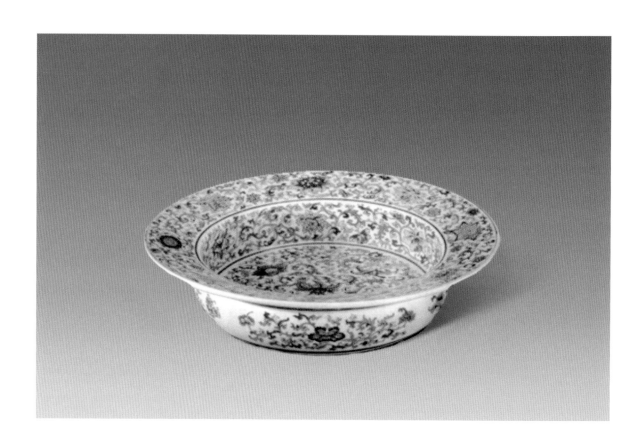

斗彩缠枝西番莲纹盆

清

瓷质

口径 43.4 厘米，通高 9.4 厘米

Doucai Basin Painted with Western Lotus Patterns

Qing Dynasty

Porcelain

Mouth Diameter 43.4 cm/ Height 9.4 cm

胎体厚重，造型大气，颇有盛世之风。宽扁的沿面斜折而出，深腹和平底庄重而稳健，底足以外的表面在金线间满施彩绘，敦厚中顿显富丽堂皇。这件乾隆时期的斗彩西番莲纹大食盆，也是中西文化交流的成果。

首都博物馆藏

The basin with thick and heavy pottery body is of grandeur and presents the flourishing empire. The wide flat rim flares out, the deep belly and flat bottom appear solemn and steady. Between two golden bowstrings on the belly there are magnificent colored patterns. The artifact, a big doucai dining basin with western lotus patterns during Qianlong Reign, was an achievement of cultural exchanges between China and western countries in the Qing Dynasty.

Preserved in the Capital Museum

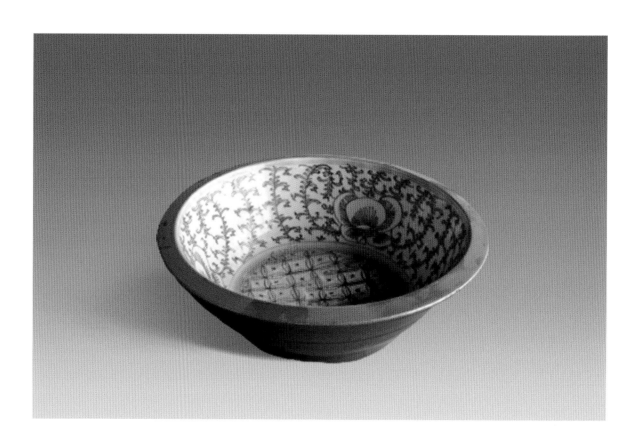

盆

清

瓷质

口径 17.5 厘米，通高 8.5 厘米

Basin

Qing Dynasty

Porcelain

Mouth Diameter 17.5 cm/ Height 8.5 cm

平口，宽沿，腹内收，平底，外壁施粉色釉，

内壁有青花缠枝纹。由民间征集。

　　成都中医药大学中医药传统文化博物馆藏

The basin has a flat mouth, wide rim, a
contracted belly, and a flat bottom. The exterior
wall is coated with pink glaze while the exterior
wall is painted with blue-and-white intertwining
floral patterns. The basin was collected from a
private owner.

Preserved in Museum of Traditional Chinese
Medicine Culture, Chengdu University of
Traditional Chinese Medicine

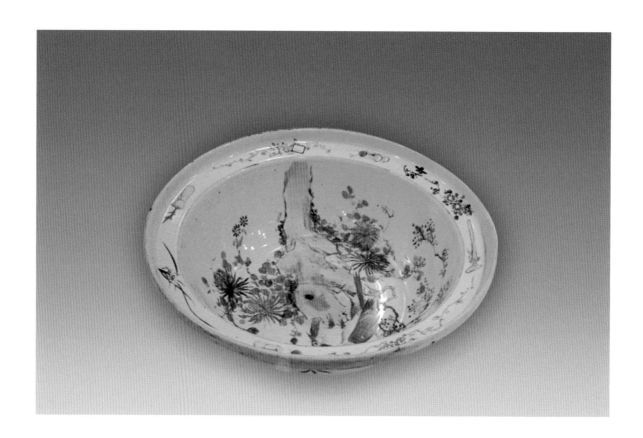

面盆

清

瓷质

口径 45 厘米，底径 28 厘米，通高 13 厘米

Basin

Qing Dynasty

Porcelain

Mouth Diameter 45 cm/ Bottom Diameter 28 cm/ Height 13 cm

直口，平肩，腹部向内倾斜，平底。饰粉彩花鸟纹，着重装饰盆底。洗面用具。由上海文物商店征集。

成都中医药大学中医药传统文化博物馆藏

The basin, which was used for face washing, has a vertical mouth, a flat shoulder, an inwardly leaning belly, and a flat bottom. It is painted with birds and flowers in famille rose palette enamel, with its bottom especially adorned. The artifact was collected from an antique shop in Shanghai.

Preserved in Museum of Traditional Chinese Medicine Culture, Chengdu University of Traditional Chinese Medicine

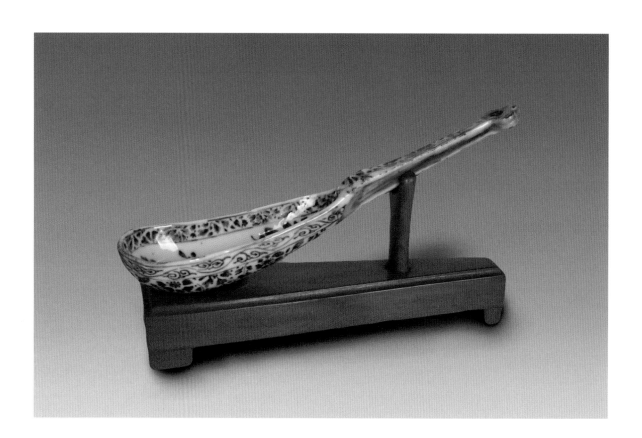

青花药洗

清

瓷质

通长 19 厘米，宽 4.1 厘米，厚 2.05 厘米

Blue-and-white Clinical Washer

Qing Dynasty

Porcelain

Length 19 cm/ Width 4.1 cm/ Thickness 2.05 cm

勺状。该藏通身施青花釉，绘有莲花莲蓬
图案，手柄为方形，柄末端有一孔，工艺
一般。为医疗用具。1957 年入藏，保存
基本完好。

中华医学会 / 上海中医药大学医史博物馆

The spoon-shaped washer, which was
for clinical use, is painted with lotus and
seedpod patterns in underglaze blue. The
rectangular parallelepiped handle has a hole
at the tapered end. The washer made with
ordinary technique was collected by the
museum in 1957 and is basically in good
condition.

Preserved in Chinese Medical Association/
Museum of Chinese Medicine, Shanghai
University of Traditional Chinese Medicine

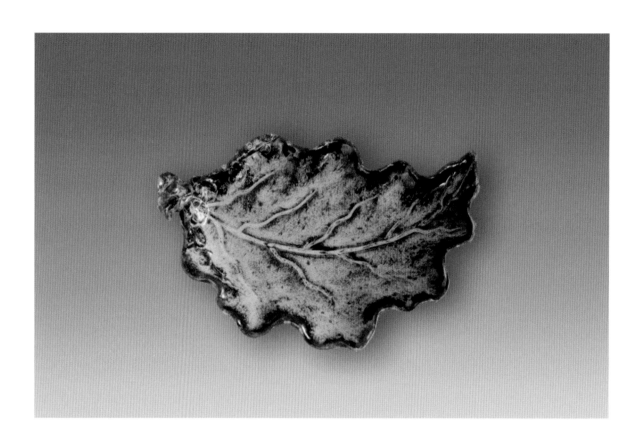

石湾窑翠毛釉秋叶洗

清

瓷质

长 25.5 厘米，宽 16.8 厘米

Autumn Leaf-shaped Brush Washer Glazed Kingfisher Blue, Shiwan Kiln

Qing Dynasty

Porcelain

Length 25.5 cm/ Width 16.8 cm

形似秋叶，平底，施棕，绿釉，莹润柔和。
石湾窑出品。

许荣坤藏

The autumn leaf-shaped brush washer has a flat bottom. It is painted with brown and green glaze which is smooth and soft. It was produced in Shiwan kiln.

Collected by Xu Rongkun

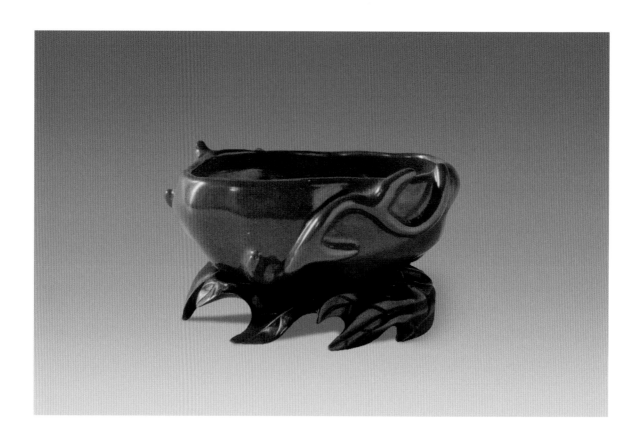

珊瑚红釉水洗

清

瓷质

口径 6.8 厘米

Coral Red-glazed Brush Washer

Qing Dynasty

Porcelain

Mouth Diameter 6.8 cm

敛口，鼓腹，形似桃形。以藤缠于桃上做装饰。施珊瑚红釉，莹润而柔和，可与天然珊瑚媲美，十分可爱。

高丰藏

The brush washer has a contracted mouth and a bulged belly like a peach with vines winding around it. The glossy and mellow coral red glaze, which coats the lovely brush-washer, can rival natural coral color.

Collected by Gao Feng

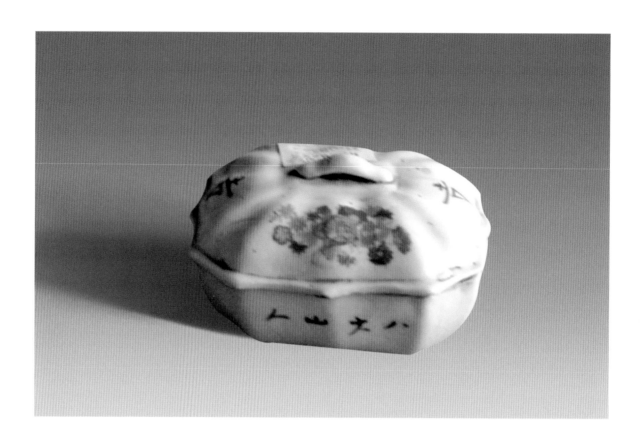

皂盒

清

瓷质

长 11 厘米，宽 9 厘米，高 7.5 厘米

Soap Box

Qing Dynasty

Porcelain

Length 11 cm/ Width 9 cm/ Height 7.5 cm

荷叶形。器盖与器身呈荷瓣形，其上绘有彩
色花卉纹饰，并墨书有"吉""寿""八大
山人"等纹，器盖上有一板桥形钮，器物造
形别致，纹饰艳丽。为日常生活中盛放皂胰
的用具。由四川省文物商店征集。

成都中医药大学中医药传统文化博物馆藏

The soap box and its lid are shaped like lotus
petal. The lid is painted with colored floral
motifs and inscribed with black ink with
Chinese words " 吉 "(Ji) (being auspicious),
" 寿 " (Shou) (longevity), and " 八 大 仙 人 "
(Ba Da Shan Ren), a prominent calligrapher
and painter who lived between the late Ming
Dynasty and the early Qing Dynasty. There
is a slab bridge-shaped knob on the lid. The
uniquely-shaped box with gorgeous patterns
was used to keep soap. It was collected from the
antique shop in Sichuan Province.
Preserved in Museum of Traditional Chinese
Medicine Culture, Chengdu University of
Traditional Chinese Medicine

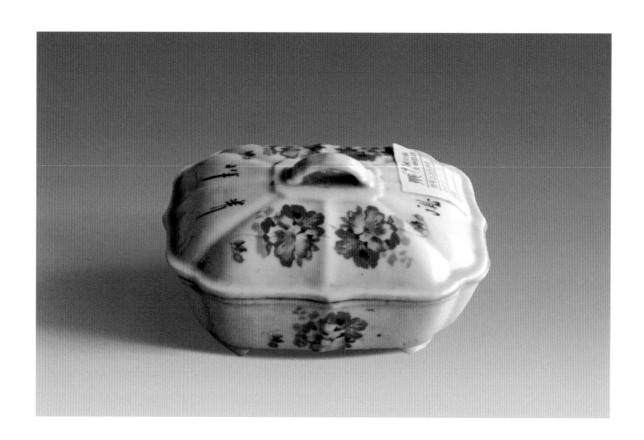

皂盒

清

瓷质

长 11 厘米，宽 9 厘米，高 7 厘米

Soap Box

Qing Dynasty

Porcelain

Length 11 cm/ Width 9 cm/ Height 7 cm

器身呈荷瓣状的鼎形，平口，腹微敛，平底，四个弧形足，内底有六个圆椎状凸起，饰彩色花卉纹，桥形纽。由四川省文物商店征集。

成都中医药大学中医药传统文化博物馆藏

The soap box shaped like a lotus petal has a flat mouth, a slightly contracted belly, a flat bottom, and four arc feet. On the lid there is a bridge-shaped knob. The interior base is formed as six cone-shaped protrusions. The artifact painted with colored floral motifs was collected from the antique shop in Sichuan Province.

Preserved in Museum of Traditional Chinese Medicine Culture, Chengdu University of Traditional Chinese Medicine

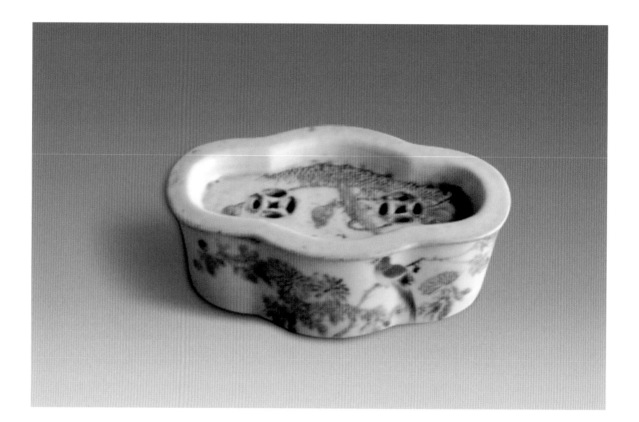

皂盒

清

瓷质

长 12.5 厘米，宽 7.5 厘米，高 4.5 厘米

Soap Box

Qing Dynasty

Porcelain

Length 12.5 cm/ Width 7.5 cm/ Height 4.5 cm

长方瓜棱形。直腹，平底，圈足。器身上饰
彩色花鸟纹和"秋色清华"等墨字，盖内凹
与器身相扣，上绘花卉纹，有两个镂空的圆
形万字孔。由四川省文物商店征集。

成都中医药大学中医药传统文化博物馆藏

The multi-lobed rectangular soap box has a
vertical belly, a flat bottom, and a ring foot. It
is painted with colored birds and floral motifs
and inscribed with inked Chinese characters
such as "Qiu Se Qing Hua" describing the
autumn scene. The dented cover, which fits in
the body, is also painted with floral motifs and
has two pierced circular patterns shaped like
the Chinese character " 万 " (Wan). The artifact
was collected from the antique shop in Sichuan
Province.

Preserved in Museum of Traditional Chinese
Medicine Culture, Chengdu University of
Traditional Chinese Medicine

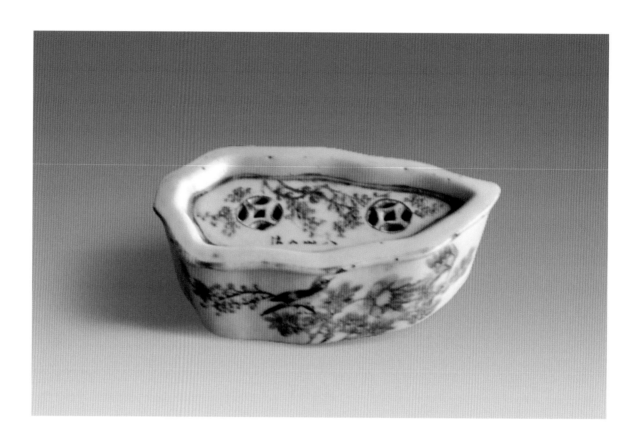

皂盒

清

瓷质

长 12.5 厘米，高 4.5 厘米

Soap Box

Qing Dynasty

Porcelain

Length 12.5 cm/ Height 4.5 cm

长方瓜棱形。直腹，平底，圈足。器身上饰彩色花鸟纹和"秋色清华"等墨字，盖内凹与器身相扣，上绘花卉纹，有两个镂空的圆形万字孔。由四川省文物商店征集。

成都中医药大学中医药传统文化博物馆藏

The multi-lobed rectangular soap box has a vertical belly, a flat bottom, and a ring foot. It is painted with colored birds and floral motifs and inscribed with inked Chinese characters such as "Qiu Se Qing Hua" describing the autumn scene. The dented cover, which fits in the body, is also painted with floral motifs and has two pierced circular patterns shaped like the Chinese character " 万 " (Wan). The artifact was collected from the antique shop in Sichuan Province.

Preserved in Museum of Traditional Chinese Medicine Culture, Chengdu University of Traditional Chinese Medicine

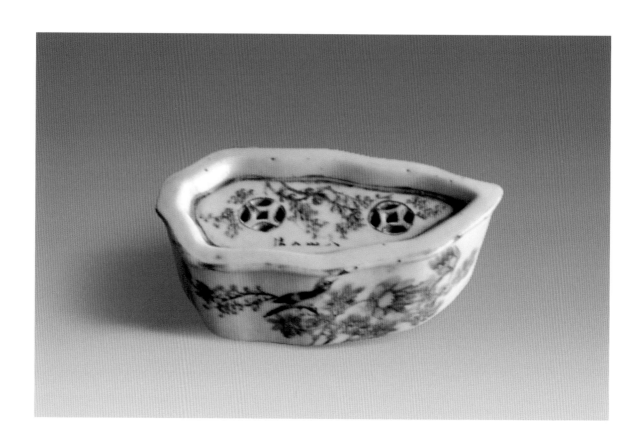

皂盒

清

瓷质

长 12.5 厘米，高 4.5 厘米

Soap Box

Qing Dynasty

Porcelain

Length 12.5 cm/ Height 4.5 cm

桃形。直口，平底，圈足。器身饰彩色花鸟纹，墨书文字，盖内凹与器身相扣，盖上饰五彩花卉纹和两个镂空圆形万字孔。由四川省文物商店征集。

成都中医药大学中医药传统文化博物馆藏

The peach-shaped soap box has a vertical mouth, a flat bottom, and a ring foot. It is painted with colored birds and floral motifs and inscribed with ink characters. The hollowed and dented cover fits in the body. The cover is also painted with colored floral motifs and has two pierced circular patterns shaped like the Chinese word " 万 " (Wan). The artifact was collected from the antique shop in Sichuan Province.

Preserved in Museum of Traditional Chinese Medicine Culture, Chengdu University of Traditional Chinese Medicine

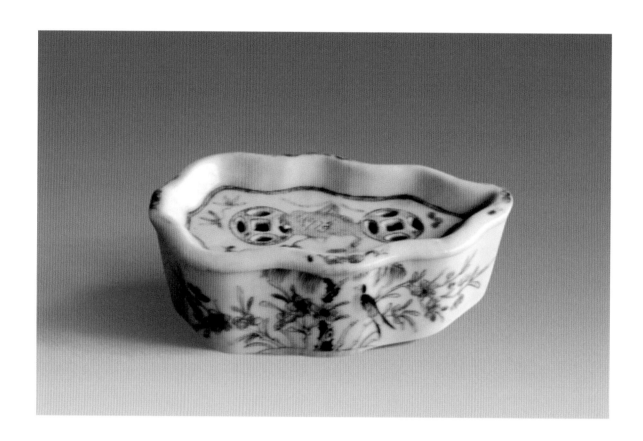

皂盒

清

瓷质

长 13 厘米，高 4.5 厘米

Soap Box

Qing Dynasty

Porcelain

Length 13 cm/ Height 4.5 cm

桃形。直口，平底，圈足。器身饰彩色花鸟纹，
盖内凹与器身相扣，盖上饰五彩花卉纹和两
个镂空圆形万字孔。由四川省文物商店征集。

　成都中医药大学中医药传统文化博物馆藏

The peach-shaped soap box has a vertical
mouth, a flat bottom, and a ring foot. It is
painted with colored birds and floral motifs.
The hollowed and dented cover fits in the body;
it is also painted with colored floral motifs and
has two pierced circular patterns shaped like the
Chinese word " 万 ". The artifact was collected
from the antique shop in Sichuan Province.
Preserved in Museum of Traditional Chinese
Medicine Culture, Chengdu University of
Traditional Chinese Medicine

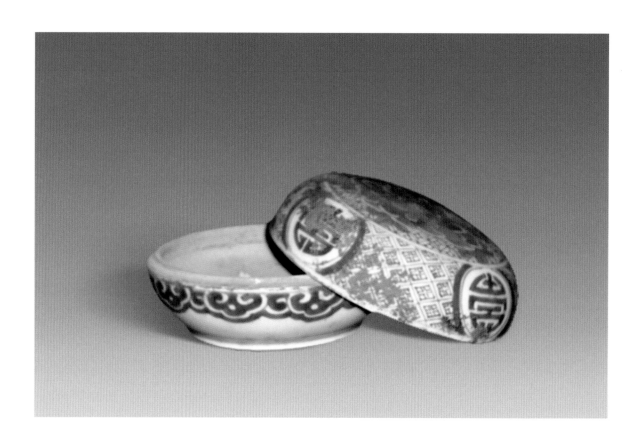

瓷盒

清

瓷质

口径 10.7 厘米，底径 7.8 厘米，通高 7 厘米，重 350 克

Porcelain Box

Qing Dynasty

Porcelain

Mouth Diameter 10.7 cm/ Bottom Diameter 7.8 cm/ Height 7 cm/ Weight 350 g

子母口，盖为半圆，盖顶牡丹花图，边有四寿字。
盛贮器。完整无损。

陕西医史博物馆藏

The box has a snap-lid. The semi-circular lid is decorated with peony motif on the top and four characteristics "Shou" (longevity) around the sides. The box was used for storage and is still in good condition.

Preserved in Shaanxi Museum of Medical History

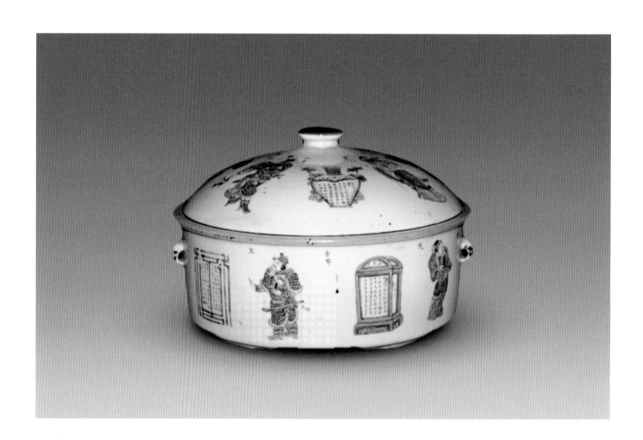

彩绘瓷盒

清

瓷质

口径 27.5 厘米，底径 25 厘米，通高 18 厘米，重 3850 克

Porcelain Box with Colored Decorations

Qing Dynasty

Porcelain

Mouth Diameter 27.5 cm/ Bottom Diameter 25 cm/ Height 18 cm/ Weight 3,850 g

彩盒带盖，子母口，直腹。腹上有四个人物，有对称的双耳。盛贮器。陕西省淳化县征集。完整无损。

陕西医史博物馆藏

The box has a lid, a mouth for a cluster mouth, a vertical belly with four figures painted on them, and a pair of symmetrical handles on the sides. The storage box, which was used for storage, was collected from Chunhua County, Shaanxi Province. It is well preserved.

Preserved in Shaanxi Museum of Medical History

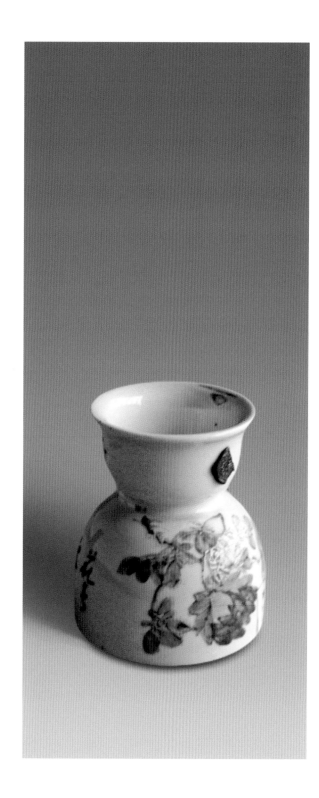

唾盂

清

瓷质

口径 7 厘米，通高 10 厘米

Spittoon

Qing Dynasty

Porcelain

Mouth Diameter 7 cm/ Height 10 cm

上下两层相连，上部敞口，鼓腹，下部为天
球形，饰有彩色花鸟纹，并墨书"花香迎春"
等字。由四川省文物商店征集。

　　成都中医药大学中医药传统文化博物馆藏

The spittoon consists of an upper part and a
lower part. The upper part has an everted mouth
and a bulged belly. The lower part, which looks
like a celestial sphere, is painted with colorful
flowers and birds and inscribed with Chinese
characters in black ink, such as "Hua Xiang
Ying Chun" (the flowers emit fragrance to
welcome the spring). The artifact was collected
from the antique store in Sichuan Province.

Preserved in Museum of Traditional Chinese
Medicine Culture, Chengdu University of
Traditional Chinese Medicine

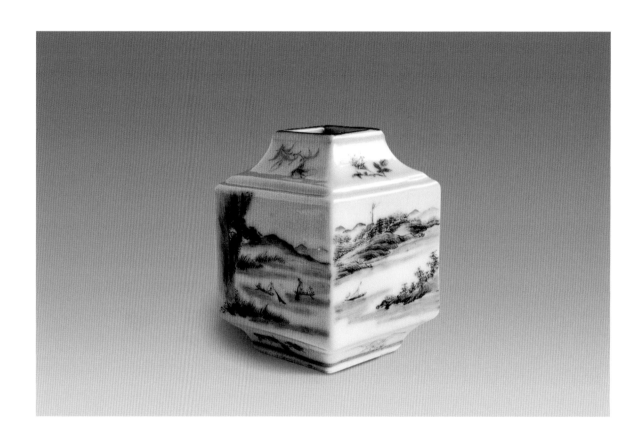

粉彩山水四方水盂

清·光绪

瓷质

口径 2 厘米，底径 3.5 厘米，通高 7 厘米

Square Water Jar Painted with Landscape in Famille Rose

Guangxu Reign, Qing Dynasty

Porcelain

Mouth Diameter 2 cm/ Bottom Diameter 3.5 cm/ Height 7 cm

该水盂成四方形，口缘和近脚处绘折枝花卉，腹的四壁绘山水纹。绘画工细，彩色鲜艳，底用矾红书写"大清光绪年制"六字楷书款。

黄卓文藏

The square water jar is painted with plucked flower branches on the mouth rim and near the foot and landscape on the four sides. The paintings are delicate and the colors are bright. The bottom is inscribed with six regular-script words "Da Qing Guang Xu Nian Zhi" (made during Guangxu Reign of the Qing Dynasty) in alum red.

Collected by Huang Zhuowen

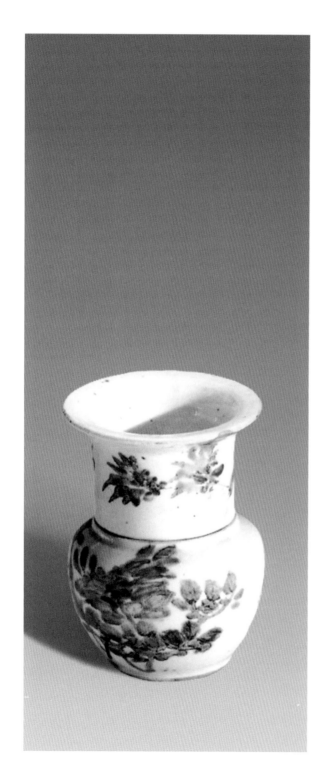

瓷唾盂

清

瓷质

口径 7.6 厘米，通高 9.8 厘米

Porcelain Spittoon

Qing Dynasty

Porcelain

Mouth Diameter 7.6 cm/ Height 9.8 cm

敞口，直颈，鼓腹，平底。上杯下盂可分开，
小巧玲珑，便于手执，方便实用。

　　成都中医药大学中医药传统文化博物馆藏

The spittoon has an everted mouth, a vertical
neck, a bugled belly, and a flat bottom. It
consists of a cup in the upper part and a
receptacle in the lower part, which can be
separated. The small and delicate spittoon
makes it easy to hold and convenient to use.

Preserved in Museum of Traditional Chinese
Medicine Culture, Chengdu University of
Traditional Chinese Medicine

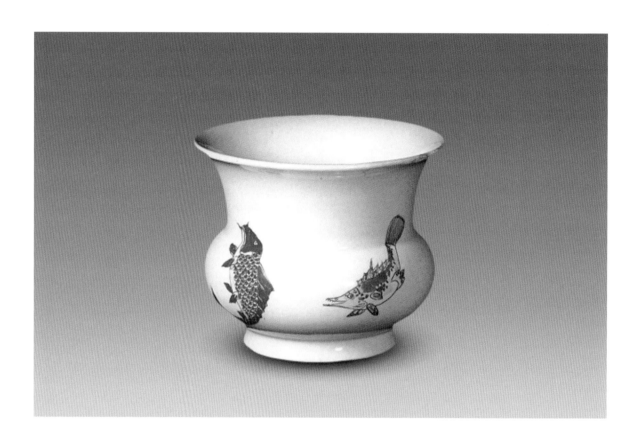

红釉四鱼唾盂

清

瓷质

底径 8 厘米，通高 12 厘米

Red-glazed Spittoon with Four Fishes

Qing Dynasty

Porcelain

Bottom Diameter 8 cm/ Height 12 cm

敞口，直鼓腹，圈足。朱绘鱼纹，形态各式，

种类不同。

上海中医药博物馆藏

The spittoon has an everted mouth, a vertical
and bulged body, and a ring foot. It is painted
with patterns of red fish of various forms and
types.

Preserved in Shanghai Museum of Traditional
Chinese Medicine

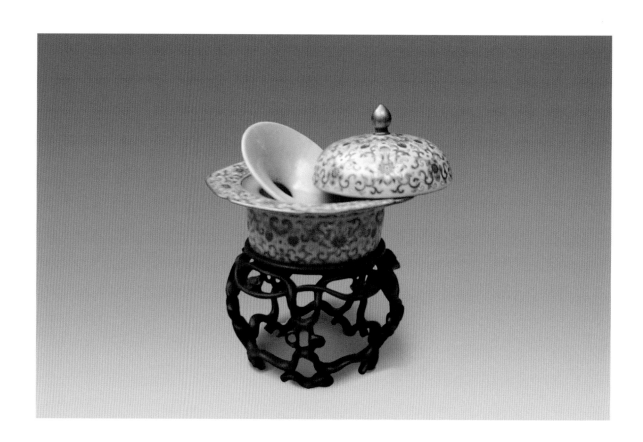

唾盂

清

瓷质

宽 14.9 厘米，通高 8.6 厘米

Spittoon

Qing Dynasty

Porcelain

Width 14.9 cm/ Height 8.6 cm

盂形。该藏通身粉彩细花，仿铜胎，平底圈足配同色盖，内置青瓷漏斗，工艺佳，造型美。为卫生用具。1959 年入藏，保存基本完好。

中华医学会 / 上海中医药大学医史博物馆

The spittoon is a broad-mouthed sanitary utensil. Its porcelain body, which looks as if it were made of copper, is painted with tiny floral patterns in famille rose. The spittoon has a flat bottom, a ring foot, and a lid glazed with the same color as the body. A celadon funnel is placed inside. The artifact, which has excellent workmanship and beautiful styling. was collected by the museum in 1959 and is basically in good condition.

Preserved in Chinese Medical Association/ Museum of Chinese Medicine, Shanghai University of Traditional Chinese Medicine

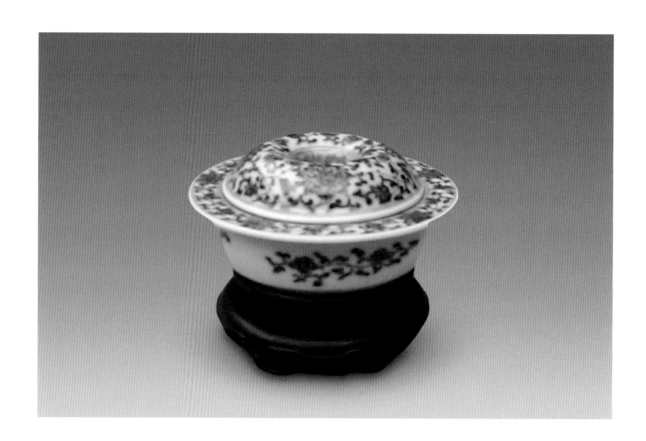

唾盂

清

瓷质

宽 12.7 厘米，通高 6 厘米

Spittoon

Qing Dynasty

Porcelain

Width 12.7 cm/ Height 6 cm

盂形。该藏青花花草图案，润泽光洁，平底，上盖有漏斗形导盂孔，工艺精良，造型美。为卫生用具。1959 年入藏，保存基本完好。

中华医学会 / 上海中医药大学医史博物馆

The spittoon is a broad-mouthed sanitary utensil. Painted with blue-and-white flower and grass patterns, it is glossy. It has a flat bottom and a lid with a funnel-shaped hole to guide spitting. The artifact is excellent in workmanship and beautiful in styling. It was collected by the museum in 1959 and is basically in good condition.

Preserved in Chinese Medical Association/ Museum of Chinese Medicine, Shanghai University of Traditional Chinese Medicine

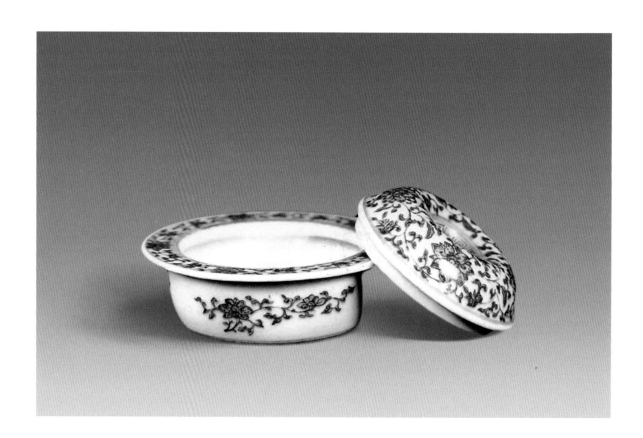

青花瓷唾盂

清

瓷质

口径 9 厘米，底径 7.2 厘米，通高 6.5 厘米

Blue-and-white Porcelain Spittoon

Qing Dynasty

Porcelain

Mouth Diameter 9 cm/ Bottom Diameter 7.2 cm/ Height 6.5 cm

此盂上下可分开，上部制成圆环状，便于使用。子母口，平底圈足，直腹，盖上有漏斗形盂孔。卫生用具。

上海中医药博物馆藏

The spittoon consists of two parts that can be separated. The upper part is shaped like a circular ring, making it convenient for use. The spittoon has a flat bottom, a ring foot, a vertical belly, and a lid with funnel-shaped hole. It was used as a sanitary utensil.

Preserved in Shanghai Museum of Traditional Chinese Medicine

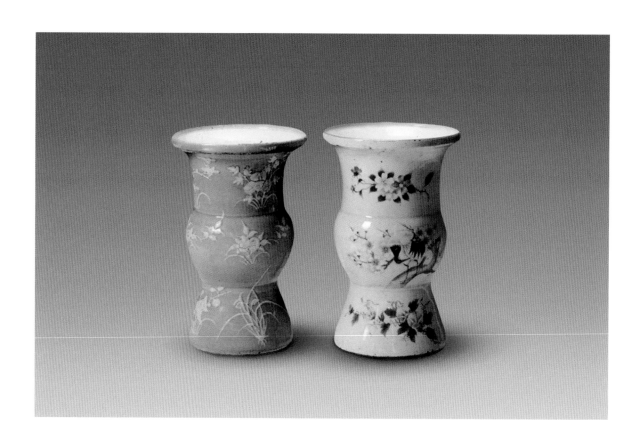

高足痰盂

清

瓷质

口径 21.5 厘米，通高 32.5 厘米

High-footed Spittoons

Qing Dynasty

Porcelain

Mouth Diameter 21.5 cm/ Height 32.5 cm

盘口，直颈，圆腰，下接喇叭型圈足，一为豆青釉，一为花卉。

成都中医药大学中医药传统文化博物馆藏

The spittoons have a plate-shaped mouth, a vertical neck, a round waist, and a trumpet-shaped bottom. One spittoon is glazed bean green while the other is decorated with flowers.

Preserved in Museum of Traditional Chinese Medicine Culture, Chengdu University of Traditional Chinese Medicine

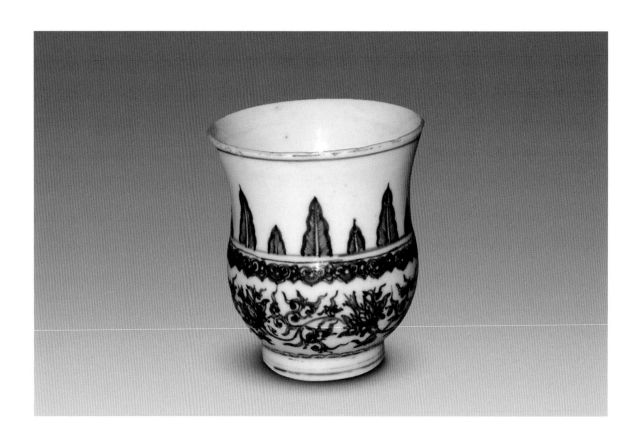

唾盂

清

瓷质

口径 11 厘米，底径 6 厘米，通高 10.8 厘米

Spittoon

Qing Dynasty

Porcelain

Mouth Diameter 11 cm/ Bottom Diameter 6 cm/ Height 10.8 cm

盂形。圈足，平底，敞口。该藏青花釉，

绘花草缠枝纹，工艺一般。卫生用具。

1959 年入藏，保存基本完好。

中华医学会 / 上海中医药大学医史博物馆

The spittoon is a broad-mouthed sanitary utensil. It has an everted mouth, a flat bottom, and a ring foot. It is painted with flower and scroll patterns in underglaze blue. The spittoon, which is ordinary in workmanship, was collected by the museum in 1959 and is basically in good condition.

Preserved in Chinese Medical Association/ Museum of Chinese Medicine, Shanghai University of Traditional Chinese Medicine

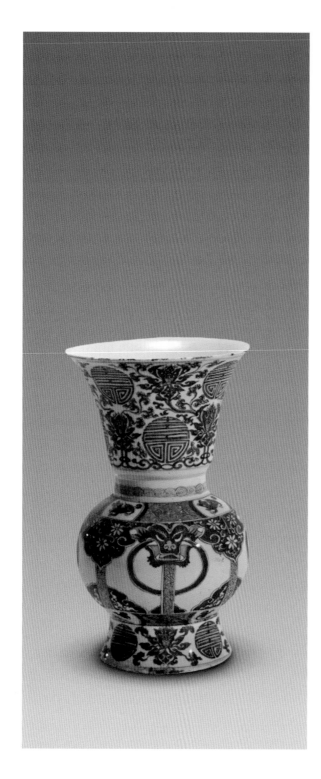

青花花觚

清

瓷质

口径 22.7 厘米，腹径 21 厘米，底径 16.5 厘米，

通高 35 厘米

Blue-and-white Porcelain Gu Vessel

Qing Dynasty

Porcelain

Mouth Diameter 22.7 cm/ Belly Diameter 21 cm/

Bottom Diameter 16.5 cm/ Height 35 cm

敞口，鼓腹。口沿微残。造型与唾盂相似。

　成都中医药大学中医药传统文化博物馆藏

The vessel has an everted mouth and a bulged belly. Its mouth rim is slightly damaged. The shape of the vessel resembles that of a spittoon.

Preserved in Museum of Traditional Chinese Medicine Culture, Chengdu University of Traditional Chinese Medicine

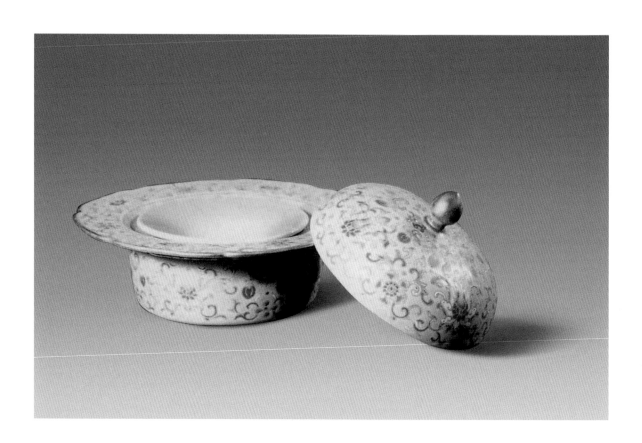

粉彩唾壶

清

瓷质

口径 7.5 厘米，底径 9 厘米，通高 9.6 厘米

Famille Rose-painted Spittoon

Qing Dynasty

Porcelain

Mouth Diameter 7.5 cm/ Bottom Diameter 9 cm/ Height 9.6 cm

上覆盖，中间隔一圆孔的喇叭形口，绿釉。外
部布满莲花卷草等勾金彩色花纹，工巧精细。

上海中医药博物馆藏

The green-glazed spittoon has a lid and a round
trumpet-shaped mouth at its center. Its surface
is decorated with lotus and scroll patterns with
golden outlines. The spittoon shows delicate
workmanship.

Preserved in Shanghai Museum of Traditional
Chinese Medicine

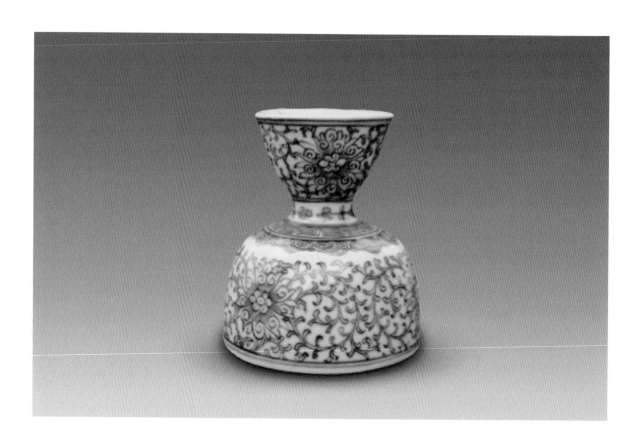

青花宝相花纹唾壶

清

瓷质

口外径 6.05 厘米，底径 8.86 厘米，腹深 9.4 厘米，通高 9.78 厘米，重 225 克

Blue-and-white Spittoon with Rosette Patterns

Qing Dynasty

Porcelain

Mouth Outer Diameter 6.05 cm/ Bottom Diameter 8.86 cm/ Belly Depth 9.4 cm/ Height 9.78 cm/ Weight 225 g

瓷质青花，盘口小，细短颈。卫生用品。

广东中医药博物馆藏

The blue-and-white porcelain spittoon has a small mouth and a short and narrow neck. It was a sanitary utensil.

Preserved in Guangdong Chinese Medicine Museum

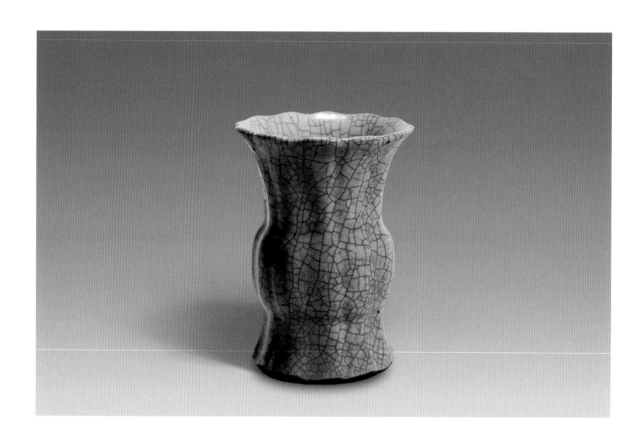

仿哥窑开片花觚

清

瓷质

口径 18.5 厘米，底径 14.5 厘米，通高 24 厘米

Decorated Gu Vessel in Copied Ge-style Glaze

Qing Dynasty

Porcelain

Mouth Diameter 18.5 cm/ Bottom Diameter 14.5 cm/ Height 24 cm

口沿莲瓣状，体部圆形多棱，器形典雅。造型
与唾盂相似。

成都中医药大学中医药传统文化博物馆藏

The gu vessel has a lotus petal-shaped mouth rim,
a round polygonal body, and elegant styling. The
shape resembles that of a spittoon.
Preserved in Museum of Traditional Chinese
Medicine Culture, Chengdu University of
Traditional Chinese Medicine

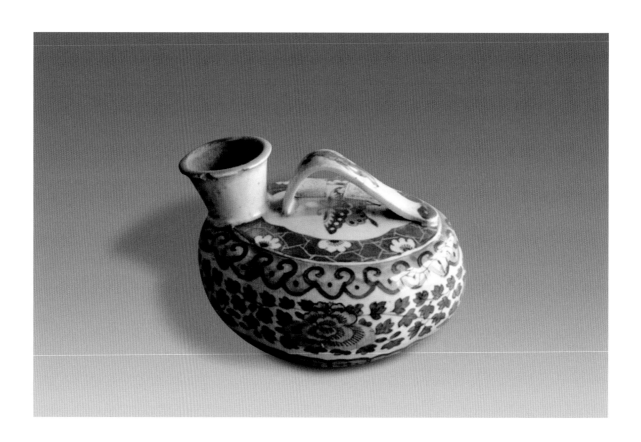

虎子

清

瓷质

长 21 厘米，宽 10 厘米

Tiger-shaped Chamber Pot

Qing Dynasty

Porcelain

Length 21 cm/ Width 10 cm

器身呈圆鼓六棱形，板桥形把，口较大，平底，器身有青花纹饰。由民间征集。

成都中医药大学中医药传统文化博物馆藏

The chamber pot has a relatively big mouth and a flat bottom. The hexagonal body, painted with patterns in underglaze blue, has bulged sides and a slab bridge-shaped handle. The pot was collected from a private owner.

Preserved in Museum of Traditional Chinese Medicine Culture, Chengdu University of Traditional Chinese Medicine

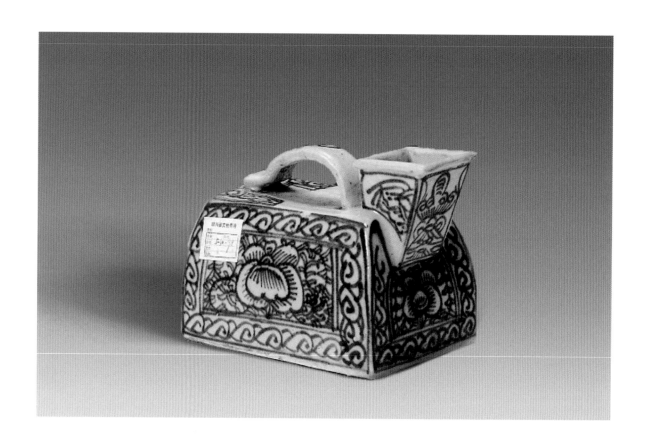

青花瓷虎子

清

瓷质

长 19 厘米，宽 12.5 厘米，高 14.5 厘米

Blue-and-white Tiger-shaped Porcelain Chamber Pot

Qing Dynasty

Porcelain

Length 19 cm/ Width 12.5 cm/ Height 14.5 cm

其口、提梁、腹部均呈方形，与通常所见虎子相左，别具一格。

　　成都中医药大学中医药传统文化博物馆藏

The mouth, handle, and body of the chamber pot are all square in shape. It has a distinctive style.

Preserved in Museum of Traditional Chinese Medicine Culture, Chengdu University of Traditional Chinese Medicine

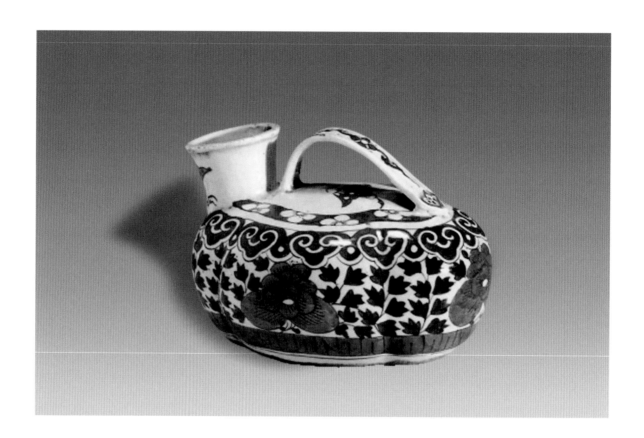

清花瓷虎子

清

瓷质

长 22 厘米，宽 17 厘米，高 16 厘米

Blue-and-white Tiger-shaped Porcelain Chamber Pot

Qing Dynasty

Porcelain

Length 22 cm/ Width 17 cm/ Height 16 cm

圆口外撇，腹部呈瓜棱型，瓷质及造型均佳。

成都中医药大学中医药传统文化博物馆藏

The chamber pot has a round and everted mouth and a ridged body. Both its porcelain quality and modeling are excellent.

Preserved in Museum of Traditional Chinese Medicine Culture, Chengdu University of Traditional Chinese Medicine

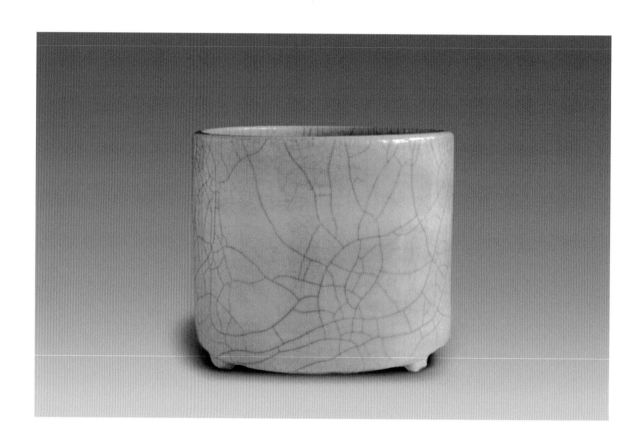

仿官窑釉直身炉

清

瓷质

口径 23 厘米，通高 19 厘米

Straight-sided Stove with Copied Official-style Glaze

Qing Dynasty

Porcelain

Mouth Diameter 23 cm/ Height 19 cm

直口，筒身，底附三足，里外满施粉青色釉，开大小纹片，黑黄相间，名为金丝铁线。釉色莹润青翠。

叶耀藏

The cylindrical stove has a vertical mouth and three feet. It is covered with powdered cyan glaze, from which can be seen big black crackles and small yellow crackles called gold thread and iron wire. The glaze is mellow and freshly green.

Collected by Ye Yao

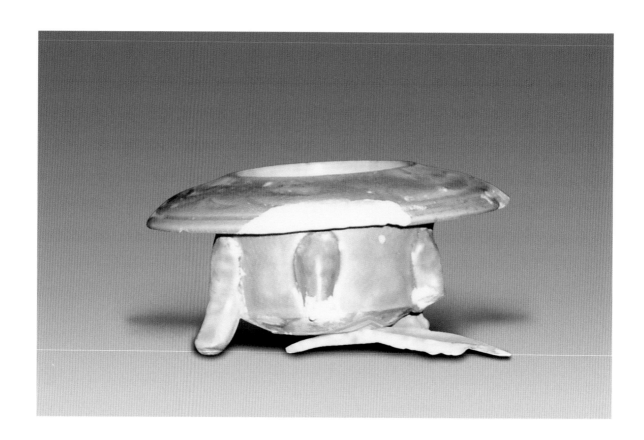

青釉五足瓷炉

清

瓷质

口径 5.5 厘米，底径 5.5 厘米，通高 5 厘米，重 100 克

Five-footed Porcelain Stove Glazed Cyan

Qing Dynasty

Porcelain

Mouth Diameter 5.5 cm/ Bottom Diameter 5.5 cm/ Height 5 cm/ Weight 100 g

圆口，平口沿，口沿上有云纹，直腹，五足。
生活用器。陕西省铜川征集。有修补。

陕西医史博物馆藏

The five-footed stove, which was for daily use, has a round mouth, a flat mouth rim with cloud patterns on it, and a vertical belly. It was collected from Tongchuan City, Shaanxi Province and has been repaired.

Preserved in Shaanxi Museum of Medical History

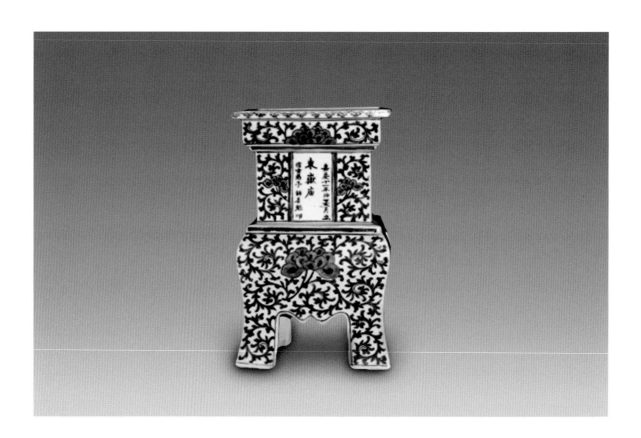

瓷香炉

清

瓷质

口径 19.4 厘米，底长 19 厘米，宽 13 厘米，通高 31.3 厘米，重 3800 克

Porcelain Incense Burner

Qing Dynasty

Porcelain

Mouth Diameter 19.4 cm/ Base Length 19 cm/ Width 13 cm/ Height 31.3 cm/ Weight 3,800 g

方盘，直颈，腹有二穿，四个三角足。祭器。

山西省张克恭征集。完整无损。

陕西医史博物馆藏

The incense burner has a rectangular mouth, a vertical neck, and four triangular feet. The sacrificial utensil collected by Zhang Kegong of Shanxi Province is still in good condition.

Preserved in Shaanxi Museum of Medical History

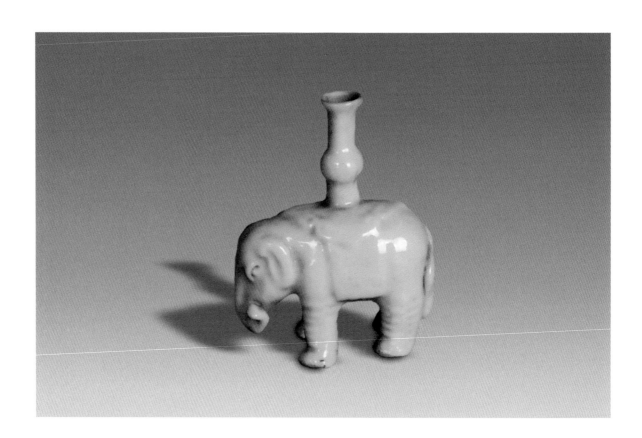

瓷香插座

清

瓷质

插口内径 0.35 厘米，插口外径 1 厘米，宽 4.4 厘米，厚 2.4 厘米，高 5.8 厘米

Porcelain Incense Holder

Qing Dynasty

Porcelain

Mouth Inner Diameter 0.35 cm/ Mouth Outer Diameter 1 cm/ Width 4.4 cm/ Thickness 2.4 cm/ Height 5.8 cm

象形。该藏通身施白釉，形似大象，象背
上竖起一香插，造型美观，工艺较好。为
插香用具。1956 年入藏。保存基本完好。

中华医学会 / 上海中医药大学医史博物馆

The white-glazed incense holder looks like an
elephant with a holder on its back. It has good
workmanship and beautiful modeling. The
artifact was collected by the museum in 1956
and is basically in good condition.
Preserved in Chinese Medical Association/
Museum of Chinese Medicine, Shanghai
University of Traditional Chinese Medicine

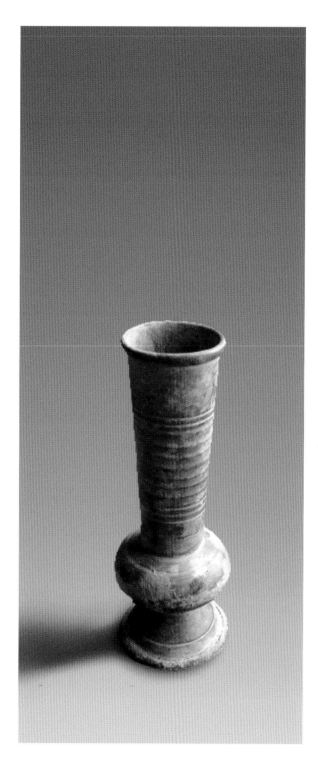

香筒

清

陶质

口径 4.5 厘米，腹宽 7 厘米，高 17.5 厘米，

Incense Pot

Qing Dynasty

Pottery

Mouth Diameter 4.5 cm/ Belly Width 7 cm/ Height

17.5 cm

敞口，长颈微收至腹，溜肩，鼓腹，平底，圈足，底部敞开。颈、腹、足上皆有旋纹，器身光滑细腻，简朴大方。香筒是古代净化空气的一种室内用具，亦可用于祭祀。

江苏省中医药博物馆藏

The pot has a flared mouth, a long neck that slightly tapers to the belly, a sloping shoulder, a bulged belly, a ring foot, and a flat and open bottom. Its neck, belly and foot are all decorated with spiral lines wile its body is smooth and simple. In ancient times the incense pot was a device used indoors to purify air and also served as a sacrificial utensil.

Preserved in Jiangsu Museum of Traditional Chinese Medicine

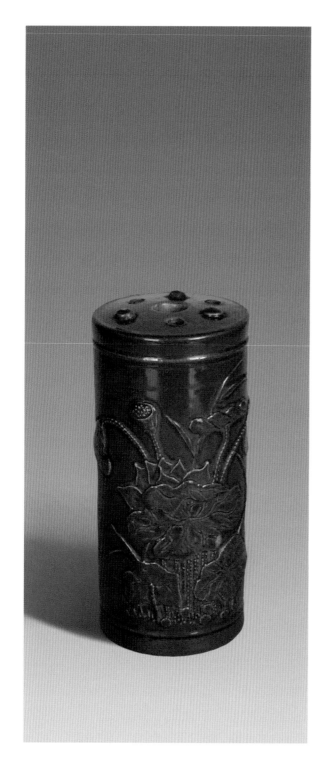

酱色瓷香筒

清

瓷质

筒径 5.4 厘米，通高 12 厘米

Porcelain Incense Pot Glazed Dark Reddish Brown

Qing Dynasty

Porcelain

Diameter 5.4 cm/ Height 12 cm

圆筒形。该藏为酱色釉，表面有荷叶莲花莲蓬图案，筒上端有一大孔和三个插香用小孔及三个小乳钉钮，做工精细。底面有"王炳榮作"款识。为香具。1957 年入藏，保存基本完好。

中华医学会 / 上海中医药大学医史博物馆

The cylindrical incense pot is glazed dark reddish brown and embossed with patterns of lotus, lotus leaves and seedpods. On its top there are a big hole, three small holes for holding joss sticks, and three tiny nipple nails. The bottom is inscribed with four Chinese characters "Wang Bingrong Zuo" (made by Wang Bingrong). The exquisite incense pot was collected by the museum in 1957 and is basically in good condition.

Preserved in Chinese Medical Association/ Museum of Chinese Medicine, Shanghai University of Traditional Chinese Medicine

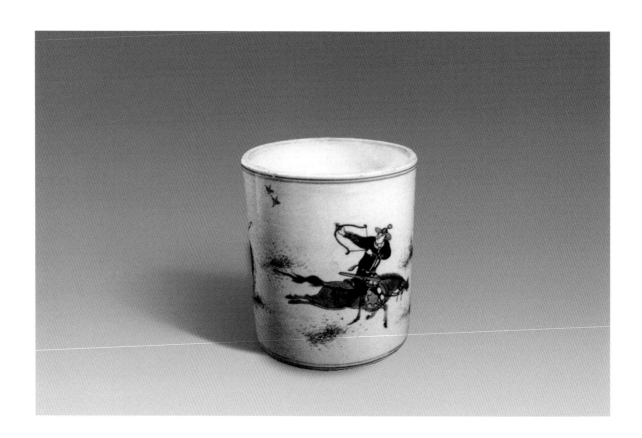

骑射纹青花瓷笔筒

清

瓷质

直径 15 厘米，高 25 厘米

Blue-and-white Porcelain Brush Pot Painted with a Man on Horse Shooting Arrow

Qing Dynasty

Porcelain

Diameter 15 cm/ Height 25 cm

笔筒为直筒形，矮圈足，口底相若。筒壁饰
有青花骑射纹，一骑士身着铠甲，头戴盔，
骑在奔驰的骏马上，正作回首弯弓而射状。

中国体育博物馆藏

The cylindrical brush pot has a short ring foot
of the similar size of the mouth. The exterior
is painted with a rider wearing an armor and
a crest who is turning his head back on a
galloping horse, about to shoot an arrow.

Preserved in China Sports Museum

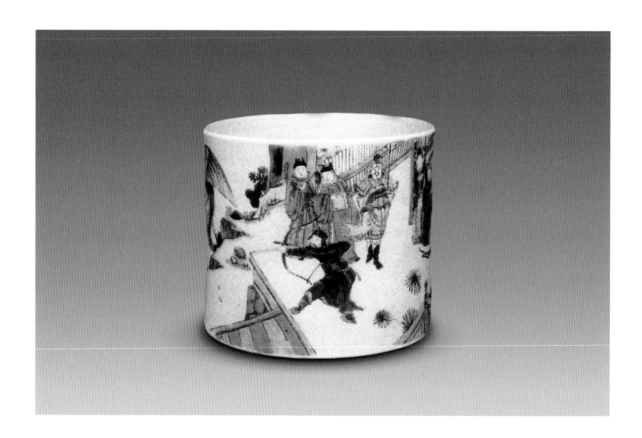

习射纹五彩瓷笔筒

清

瓷质

高 16.3 厘米

Five-colored Porcelain Brush Pot with Shooting Practice Scene

Qing Dynasty

Porcelain

Height 16.3 cm

直筒形。胎质洁白细腻，釉质晶莹匀净。图画用
五彩描绘了以射箭活动为主的人物形象，个个神
态迥异，其中的射箭者正弓腿曲身作欲射状。画
面中的人物神情和动作表现得淋漓尽致。

法国吉美国立亚洲艺术博物馆藏

The cylindrical brush pot has pure white and fine
pottery body and glossy and homogeneous glaze. The
five-colored painting on the exterior mainly depicts
a figure shooting an arrow: the shooter, with his
legs and his back bent, is ready to shoot; the facial
expressions and movements that differ from one
person to another are lively and real.

Preserved in Musée National des Arts Asiatiques-
Guimet, France

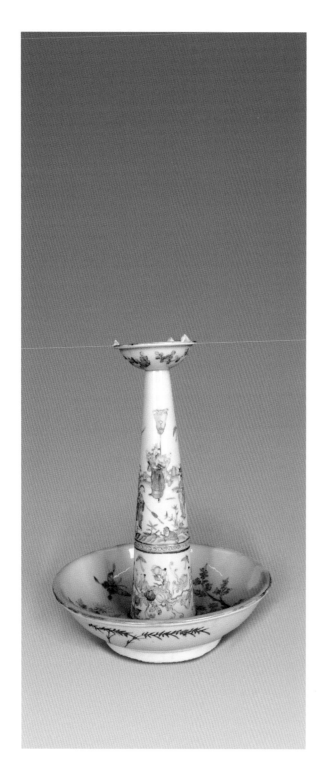

油灯

清

瓷质

宽 23.4 厘米，通高 27.7 厘米

Oil Lamp

Qing Dynasty

Porcelain

Width 23.4 cm/ Height 27.7 cm

灯盏形。该藏粉彩釉，绘人物故事图案，

假圈足，空心柱，下部托盘，造型美观。

灯具。1955年入藏，保存基本完好。

中华医学会/上海中医药大学医史博物馆

The beautifully-shaped oil lamp is glazed famille rose and painted with stories of figures. It has a false ring foot, a hollow pillar, and a stand. It was collected by the museum in 1955 and is basically in good condition.

Preserved in Chinese Medical Association/ Museum of Chinese Medicine, Shanghai University of Traditional Chinese Medicine

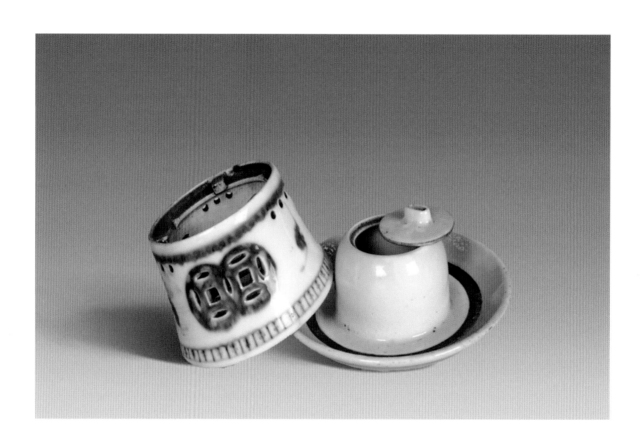

油灯

清

瓷质

宽 15.5 厘米，通高 8.7 厘米

Oil Lamp

Qing Dynasty

Porcelain

Width 15.5 cm/ Height 8.7 cm

灯形。该藏青花釉，有托盘连油缸、油灯嘴和灯罩组成，灯罩上有三组镂空双钱图案和三只蝙蝠，沿口处有九小孔亦分三组，圈足平底，盘底绘乡间风景画，造型考究。灯具。1956 年入藏，保存基本完好。

中华医学会 / 上海中医药大学医史博物馆

The blue-and-white porcelain lamp that is exquisitely shaped consists of a stand, an oil cylinder, a lampmouth, and a lampshade. The lamp has a ring foot and a flat bottom which is painted with rural landscape. The lampshade is painted with three bats and pierced with three pairs of coin patterns. There are three groups of small holes near the mouth rim. The lamp was collected by the museum in 1956 and is basically in good condition.

Preserved in Chinese Medical Association/ Museum of Chinese Medicine, Shanghai University of Traditional Chinese Medicine

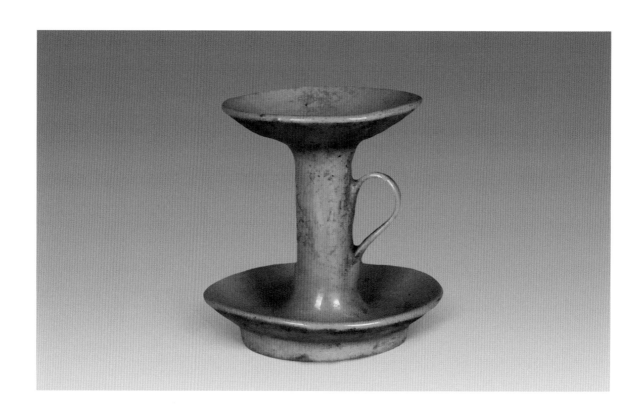

瓷油灯

清

瓷质

宽 10.2 厘米，高 10.1 厘米

Porcelain Oil Lamp

Qing Dynasty

Porcelain

Width 10.2 cm/ Height 10.1 cm

灯盏形。该藏施绿釉，由上油碟和下托盘

组成，中部有桥状把手，圈足空心底无釉，

工艺一般。为灯具。1955 年入藏，保存

基本完好。

中华医学会 / 上海中医药大学医史博物馆

The green-glazed oil lamp consists of an oil
plate as the upper part, a stand as the lower
part, a bridge-shaped handle as the middle
part, and a hollowed and unglazed ring foot.
It is ordinary in workmanship. The lamp was
collected by the museum in 1955 and is
basically in good condition.
Preserved in Chinese Medical Association/
Museum of Chinese Medicine, Shanghai
University of Traditional Chinese Medicine

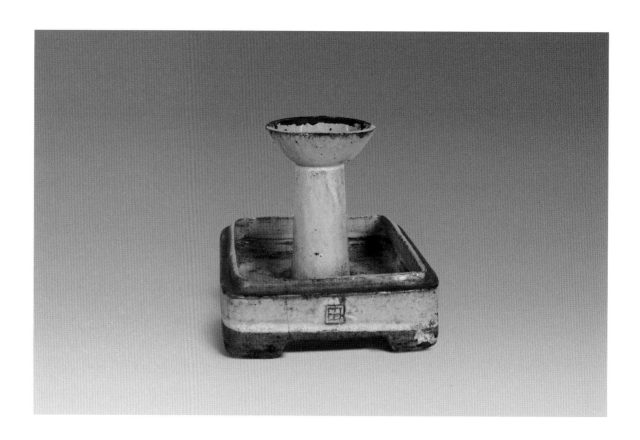

瓷风油灯

清

瓷质

方座边长 14.5 厘米，灯盏内径 6.6 厘米，灯盏外径 7.6 厘米，灯盏深 2.7 厘米，通高 13.5 厘米

Porcelain Oil Lamp

Qing Dynasty

Porcelain

Length of the Square Stand 14.5 cm/ Inner Diameter of the Oil Cup 6.6 cm/ Outer Diameter of the Oil Cup 7.6 cm/ Depth of the Oil Cup 2.7 cm/ Height 13.5 cm

灯盏形。该藏粗瓷制作，施浅黄色釉，小

开片，底座边缘釉"田"字款，工艺一般，

为灯具。1958 年入藏，保存基本完好。

　中华医学会 / 上海中医药大学医史博物馆

The lamp with tiny crackles is made of crude

porcelain glazed light yellow. The rim of its

stand is inscribed with one-word seal mark

"Tian". The lamp is ordinary in workmanship.

It was collected by the museum in 1958 and

is basically in good condition.

Preserved in Chinese Medical Association/

Museum of Chinese Medicine, Shanghai

University of Traditional Chinese Medicine

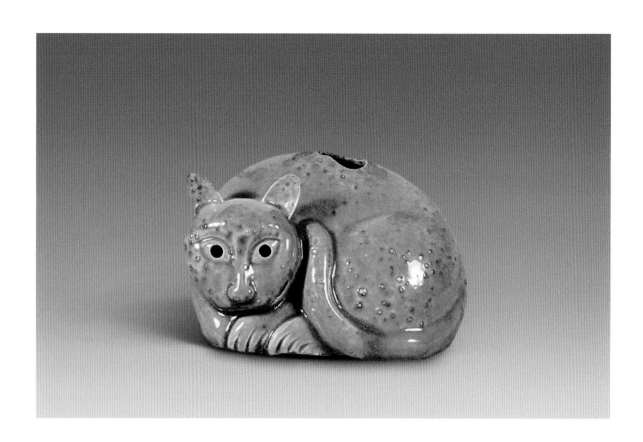

孔雀绿猫形灯

清

瓷质

宽 18 厘米，高 11.5 厘米

Peacock Green Cat-shaped Lampholder

Qing Dynasty

Width 18 cm/ Height 11.5 cm

此器内壁露胎，色灰白。猫头、尾、足均在前作盘坐式。无底中空可置油灯，竖起的耳及眼、口、背均镂空，放射出灯光。古人为保护停尸，以此灯置于尸体前，用来驱鼠。

上海中医药博物馆藏

The inner surface is grayish white without glaze. A cat's head, tail and feet are in coiling position in the front of the lampholder. An oil lamp can be placed inside the bottomless lampshade. The cat's erect ears, eyes, mouth and back are all hollowed out so that light can emit through them. Chinese people in ancient times placed this lampholder beside a corpse to keep rats away.

Preserved in Shanghai Museum of Traditional Chinese Medicine

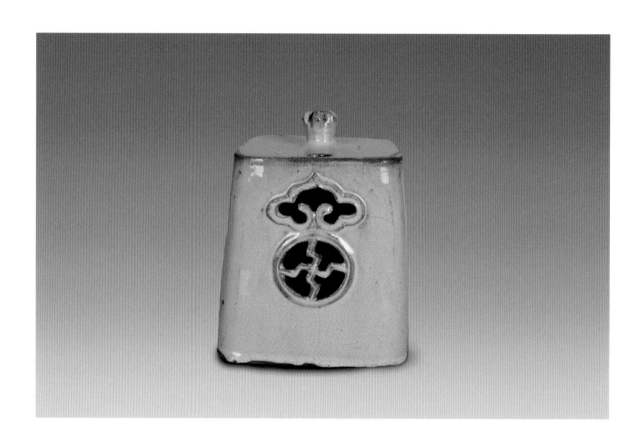

瓷风油灯罩

清

瓷质

方罩边长 14.6 厘米，通高 18.9 厘米

Porcelain Lampshade

Qing Dynasty

Porcelain

Length 14.6 cm/ Height 18.9 cm

方形。该藏粗瓷，施浅黄色釉，小开片，
罩内壁无釉，上有一孔（直径 1.6 厘米），
三面封闭，一面有镂空图案，顶端有一佛
手钮。工艺一般。为灯具。1958 年入藏，
保存基本完好。

中华医学会 / 上海中医药大学医史博物馆

The square lampshade is made of crude
porcelain with tiny crackles. The exterior
is glazed light yellow. Only one side of the
lampshade is pierced with a pattern. On the
top there is a knob shaped like Buddha's
hand, and near it there is a small hole of
1.6 cm in diameter. The lampshade has
ordinary craftsmanship. It was collected by
the museum in 1958 and is basically in good
condition.

Preserved in Chinese Medical Association/
Museum of Chinese Medicine, Shanghai
University of Traditional Chinese Medicine

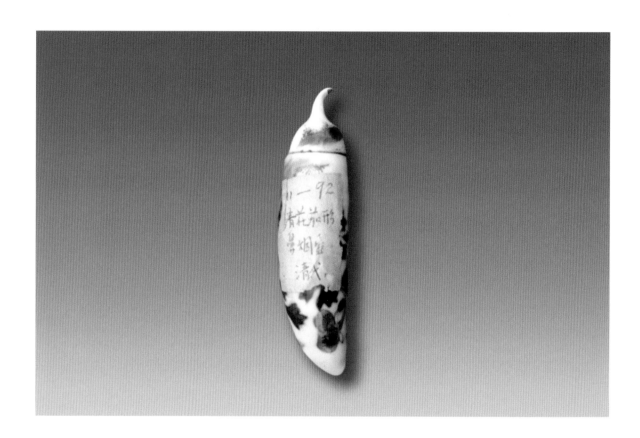

青花茄形鼻烟壶

清

瓷质

腹径 2.3 厘米，通高 8.19 厘米，重 31 克

Blue-and-white Eggplant-shaped Snuff Bottle

Qing Dynasty

Porcelain

Belly Diameter 2.3 cm/ Height 8.19 cm/ Weight 31 g

青花茄形，带盖，用于盛装鼻烟的容器。

广东中医药博物馆藏

The eggplant-shaped snuff bottle has a lid. It was used for storing snuff.

Preserved in Guangdong Chinese Medicine Museum

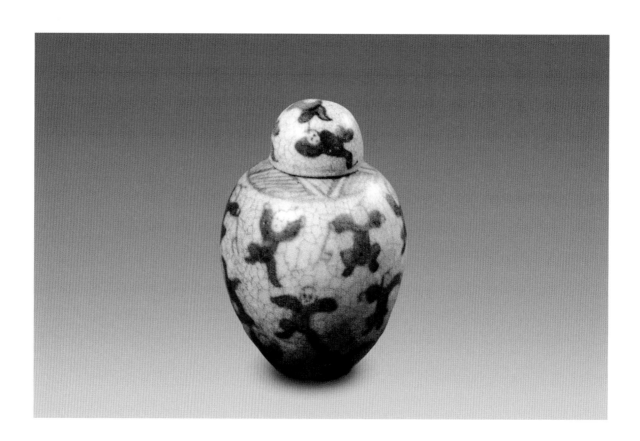

拳术演练纹青花鼻烟壶

清

瓷质

腹径 5 厘米，高 7.5 厘米

Blue-and-white Snuff Bottle with Chinese Boxing Practice Scene

Qing Dynasty

Porcelain

Belly Diameter 5 cm/ Height 7.5 cm

鼻烟壶为小口，鼓腹，平底，口上置一半圆
形盖。拳术演练纹饰于壶的腹部和盖面，从
人物演练的招式和动作看，应是一种连贯的
拳术套路动作。

中国体育博物馆藏

The snuff bottle has a small mouth with a
hemispherical lid on it, a bulged belly, and a flat
bottom. The belly and the lid are decorated with
the scene of Chinese boxing practice, which
may be a set of successive movements judging
from the figures' movements and gestures.

Preserved in China Sports Museum

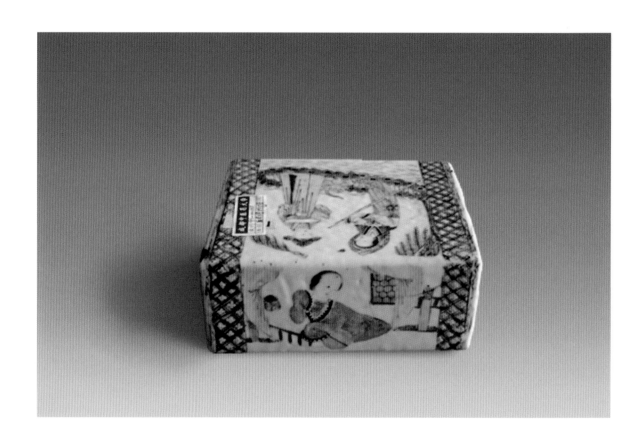

枕

清

瓷质

长 14.5 厘米，宽 12 厘米，高 6 厘米

Head-rest

Qing Dynasty

Porcelain

Length 14.5 cm/ Width 12 cm/ Height 6 cm

器身扁平，施五彩人物图案于四面，两侧有
铜线形孔，由民间征集。

成都中医药大学中医药传统文化博物馆藏

The flat head-rest has multi-colored figures on
the four sides and holes like copper line in the
rectangular ends. It was collected from a private
owner.

Preserved in Museum of Traditional Chinese
Medicine Culture, Chengdu University of
Traditional Chinese Medicine

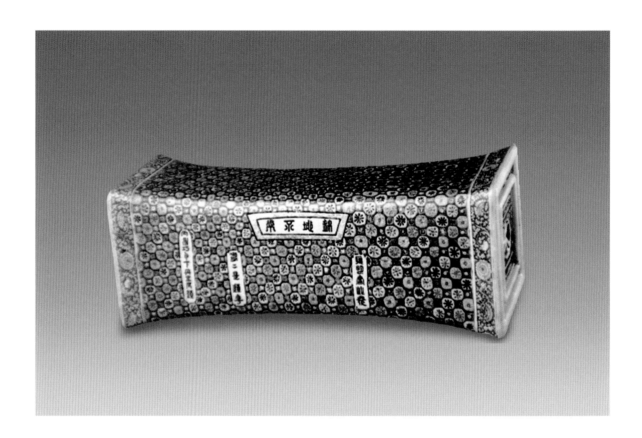

五彩描金锦地莲花纹枕

清

瓷质

长 40.8 厘米，宽 15.6 厘米，高 15.6 厘米

Famille Noire Head-rest Painted with Lotus Patterns Against Gold-depicting Brocade-like Background

Qing Dynasty

Porcelain

Length 40.8 cm/ Width 15.6 cm/ Height 15.6 cm

长方形。两头略高，中部略低，形成弧面。枕面以矾红彩锦地为主，一面锦地上有篆书题字，左为"□二是□□"，右为"聪明当此发"，横书"锦地永常"，落款为"丙□巧月卞丹主人题"。枕两头镂空。作品用心巧妙，装饰华贵，是一各种睡眠用具。

故宫博物院藏

The rectangular head-rest is higer on the two long sides but lover in the cnter, forming a curved surface. Its surface is mainly made of iron-red colored brocade. One side is inscribed with some words in seal characters. The two ends of the head-set are hollow. This artistic piece used for sleep is ingenious in design and luxurious in decoraxon.

Preserved in the Palace Museum, Beijing

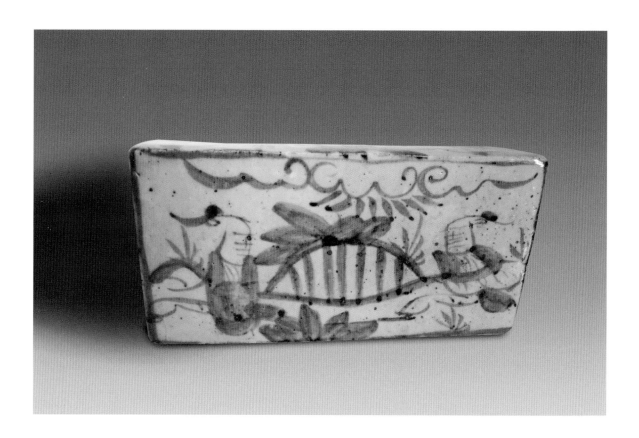

青花脉枕

清

瓷质

长 18 厘米，宽 9 厘米，高 5 厘米

Blue-and-white Porcelain Pillow Used for Pulse Taking

Qing Dynasty

Porcelain

Length 18 cm/ Width 9 cm/ Height 5 cm

长方形。脉枕是中医大夫诊脉时放在患者腕
下起衬垫作用的用具，体积很小，重量很轻，
便于携带。

新昌县天姥中医博物馆藏

The rectangular pillow was used for putting
a patient's wrist under as a cushion when a
Traditional Chinese Medicine practitioner was
taking his or her pulse. Its small size and light
weight make it easily carried around.

Preserved in Tianlao Museum of Traditional
Chinese Medicine of Xinchang County,
Zhejiang Province

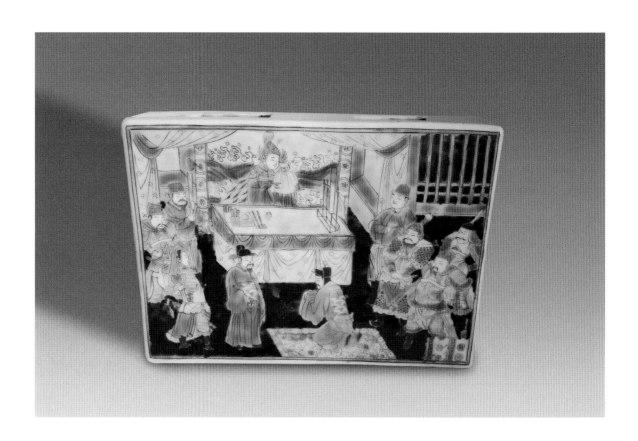

人物故事纹脉枕

清

瓷质

长 21 厘米，宽 15 厘米，高 4.2 厘米

Character-featured Pillow Used for Pulse Taking

Qing Dynasty

Porcelain

Length 21 cm/ Width 15 cm/ Height 4.2 cm

箱型。脉枕下面有两长方形小孔，它们是烧

制时为防止爆裂而设的排气孔。脉枕是中医

大夫诊脉时放在患者腕下起衬垫作用的用具，

体积很小，重量很轻，便于携带。

新昌县天姥中医博物馆藏

The case-shaped pillow has two small
rectangular holes underneath, which were used
for ventilating holes to prevent it from bursting
during baking. The pillow was used for putting
a patient's wrist under as a cushion when a
Traditional Chinese Medicine practitioner was
taking his or her pulse. Its small size and light
weight make it easily carried around.

Preserved in Tianlao Museum of Traditional
Chinese Medicine of Xinchang County,
Zhejiang Province

索 引

（馆藏地按拼音字母排序）

朱德明

庄锡忠

Index

参考文献

[1] 李经纬 . 中国古代医史图录 [M]. 北京：人民卫生出版社，1992.

[2] 傅维康，李经纬，林昭庚 . 中国医学通史：文物图谱卷 [M]. 北京：人民卫生出版社，2000.

[3] 和中浚，吴鸿洲 . 中华医学文物图集 [M]. 成都：四川人民出版社，2001.

[4] 上海中医药博物馆 . 上海中医药博物馆馆藏珍品 [M]. 上海：上海科学技术出版社，2013.

[5] 西藏自治区博物馆 . 西藏博物馆 [M]. 北京：五洲传播出版社，2005.

[6] 崔乐泉 . 中国古代体育文物图录：中英文本 [M]. 北京：中华书局，2000.

[7] 张金明，陆雪春 . 中国古铜镜鉴赏图录 [M]. 北京：中国民族摄影艺术出版社，2002.

[8] 文物精华编辑委员会 . 文物精华 [M]. 北京：文物出版社，1964.

[9] 谭维四 . 湖北出土文物精华 [M]. 武汉：湖北教育出版社，2001.

[10] 常州市博物馆 . 常州文物精华 [M]. 北京：文物出版社，1998.

[11] 镇江博物馆 . 镇江文物精华 [M]. 合肥：黄山书社，1997.

[12] 贵州省文化厅，贵州省博物馆 . 贵州文物精华 [M]. 贵阳：贵州人民出版社，2005.

[13] 徐良玉 . 扬州馆藏文物精华 [M]. 南京：江苏古籍出版社，2001.

[14] 昭陵博物馆，陕西历史博物馆 . 昭陵文物精华 [M]. 西安：陕西人民美术出版社，1991.

[15] 南通博物苑 . 南通博物苑文物精华 [M]. 北京：文物出版社，2005.

[16] 邯郸市文物研究所 . 邯郸文物精华 [M]. 北京：文物出版社，2005.

[17] 张秀生，刘友恒，聂连顺，等 . 中国河北正定文物精华 [M]. 北京：文化艺术出版社，1998.

[18] 陕西省咸阳市文物局 . 咸阳文物精华 [M]. 北京：文物出版社，2002.

[19] 安阳市文物管理局 . 安阳文物精华 [M]. 北京：文物出版社，2004.

[20] 深圳市博物馆 . 深圳市博物馆文物精华 [M]. 北京：文物出版社，1998.

[21]《中国文物精华》编辑委员会 . 中国文物精华（1993）[M]. 北京：文物出版社，1993.

[22] 夏路，刘永生. 山西省博物馆馆藏文物精华 [M]. 太原：山西人民出版社，1999.

[23] 文物精华编辑委员会. 文物精华 [M]. 北京：文物出版社，1957.

[24] 山西博物院，湖北省博物馆. 荆楚长歌：九连墩楚墓出土文物精华 [M]. 太原：山西人民出版社，2011.

[25] 刘广堂，石金鸣，宋建忠. 晋国雄风：山西出土两周文物精华 [M]. 沈阳：万卷出版公司，2009.

[26] 沈君山，王国平，单迎红. 滦平博物馆馆藏文物精华 [M]. 北京：中国文联出版社，2012.

[27] 张家口市博物馆. 张家口市博物馆馆藏文物精华 [M]. 北京：科学出版社，2011.

[28] 浙江省文物考古研究所. 浙江考古精华 [M]. 北京：文物出版社，1999.

[29] 故宫博物院. 故宫雕刻珍萃 [M]. 北京：紫禁城出版社，2004.

[30] 故宫博物院紫禁城出版社. 故宫博物院藏宝录 [M]. 上海：上海文艺出版社，1986.

[31] 首都博物馆. 大元三都 [M]. 北京：科学出版社，2016.

[32] 新疆维吾尔自治区博物馆. 新疆出土文物 [M]. 北京：文物出版社，1975.

[33] 王兴伊，段逸山. 新疆出土涉医文书辑校 [M]. 上海：上海科学技术出版社，2016.

[34] 刘学春. 刍议医药卫生文物的概念与分类标准 [J]. 中华中医药杂志，2016，31（11）:4406-4409.

[35] 上海古籍出版社. 中国艺海 [M]. 上海：上海古籍出版社，1994.

[36] 紫都，岳鑫. 一生必知的 200 件国宝 [M]. 呼和浩特：远方出版社，2005.

[37] 谭维四. 湖北出土文物精华 [M]. 武汉：湖北教育出版社，2001.

[38] 张建青. 青海彩陶收藏与鉴赏 [M]. 北京：中国文史出版社，2007.

[39] 银景琦. 仡佬族文物 [M]. 南宁：广西人民出版社，2014.

[40] 廖果，梁峻，李经纬. 东西方医学的反思与前瞻 [M]. 北京：中医古籍出版社，2002.

[41] 梁峻，张志斌，廖果，等. 中华医药文明史集论 [M]. 北京：中医古籍出版社，2003.

[42] 郑蓉，庄乾竹，刘聪，等. 中国医药文化遗产考论 [M]. 北京：中医古籍出版社，2005.